The Lymphatic System in Thoracic Oncology

Guest Editors

FEDERICO VENUTA, MD
ERINO A. RENDINA, MD

THORACIC SURGERY CLINICS

www.thoracic.theclinics.com

Consulting Editor
MARK K. FERGUSON, MD

May 2012 • Volume 22 • Number 2

SAUNDERS an imprint of ELSEVIER, Inc.

W.B. SAUNDERS COMPANY
A Division of Elsevier Inc.

1600 John F. Kennedy Boulevard • Suite 1800 • Philadelphia, Pennsylvania 19103-2899

http://www.theclinics.com

THORACIC SURGERY CLINICS Volume 22, Number 2
May 2012 ISSN 1547-4127, ISBN-13: 978-1-4557-3944-8

Editor: Barbara Cohen-Kligerman
Developmental Editor: Teia Stone

Thoracic Surgery Clinics (ISSN 1547-4127) is published quarterly by Elsevier Inc., 360 Park Avenue South, New York, NY 10010-1710. Months of publication are February, May, August, and November. Business and editorial offices: 1600 John F. Kennedy Boulevard, Suite 1800, Philadelphia, PA 19103-2899. Periodicals postage paid at New York, NY, and additional mailing offices. Subscription prices are $322.00 per year (US individuals), $416.00 per year (US institutions), $154.00 per year (US Students), $400.00 per year (Canadian individuals), $526.00 per year (Canadian institutions), $209.00 per year (Canadian and foreign students), $426.00 per year (foreign individuals), and $526.00 per year (foreign institutions). Foreign air speed delivery is included in all Clinics' subscription prices. All prices are subject to change without notice. **POSTMASTER:** Send address changes to Thoracic Surgery Clinics, Elsevier Health Sciences Division, Subscription Customer Service, 3251 Riverport Lane, Maryland Heights, MO 63043. **Customer Service (orders, claims, online, change of address): Telephone: 1-800-654-2452 (U.S. and Canada); 314-447-8871 (outside U.S. and Canada). Fax: 314-447-8029. Email: journalscustomerservice-usa@elsevier.com (for print support); journalsonlinesupport-usa@elsevier.com (for online support).**

Reprints. For copies of 100 or more, of articles in this publication, please contact Commercial Rights Department, Elsevier Inc., 360 Park Avenue South, New York, NY 10010-1710. Tel: (212) 633-3812; Fax: (212) 462-1935; E-mail: reprints@elsevier.com.

Thoracic Surgery Clinics is covered in *MEDLINE/PubMed (Index Medicus)* and *EMBASE/Excerpta Medica.*

Printed and bound by CPI Group (UK) Ltd, Croydon, CR0 4YY

Transferred to Digital Print 2012

Contributors

CONSULTING EDITOR

MARK K. FERGUSON, MD
Professor of Surgery, Section of Cardiac and
Thoracic Surgery, The University of Chicago
Medical Center, Chicago, Illinois

GUEST EDITORS

FEDERICO VENUTA, MD
Professor, Department of Thoracic Surgery,
Policlinico Umberto I; Fondazione Lorillard
Spencer-Cenci, University La Sapienza,
Rome, Italy

ERINO A. RENDINA, MD
Professor and Chief, Department of Thoracic
Surgery, Sant'Andrea Hospital, University
La Sapienza, Rome, Italy

AUTHORS

CIPRIAN BOLCA, MD
Clinical Fellow, Department of Thoracic
Surgery, Institut Universitaire de Cardiologie
et de Pneumologie de Québec (IUCPQ),
Quebec City, Quebec, Canada

GIUSEPPE BONI, MD
Doctor, Regional Center of Nuclear Medicine,
University of Pisa, Pisa, Italy

STEPHEN R. BRODERICK, MD
Instructor of Surgery, Division of
Cardiothoracic Surgery, Department of
Surgery, Washington University School of
Medicine, St. Louis, Missouri

MATIAS LOSANO BROTONS, MD
Clinical Fellow, Department of Thoracic
Surgery, Institut Universitaire de Cardiologie
et de Pneumologie de Québec (IUCPQ),
Quebec City, Quebec, Canada

AYESHA S. BRYANT, MD, MSPH
Assistant Professor, Division of Cardiothoracic
Surgery, University of Alabama at Birmingham,
Birmingham, Alabama

SERGI CALL, MD, FETCS
Attending Thoracic Surgeon, Thoracic Surgery
Service, Hospital Universitari Mutua Terrassa,
University of Barcelona, Terrassa,
Barcelona, Spain

GIUSEPPE CAMPENNÌ, MD
Medical Oncology Division, Sapienza–
University of Rome, Rome, Italy

CARLO CATALANO, MD
Professor, Department of Radiology, University
La Sapienza, Policlinico Umberto I, Rome, Italy

ROBERT J. CERFOLIO, MD
Professor, Thoracic Surgery; Section Chief,
Division of Cardiothoracic Surgery, University
of Alabama at Birmingham, Birmingham,
Alabama

DAVIDE CONTE, MD
Medical Oncology Division, Sapienza–
University of Rome, Rome, Italy

ENRICO CORTESI, MD
Medical Oncology Division, Sapienza–
University of Rome, Rome, Italy

ANTONIO D'ANDRILLI, MD
Assistant Professor of Thoracic Surgery,
Department of Thoracic Surgery, Sant'Andrea
Hospital, University La Sapienza, Rome, Italy

HIROSHI DATE, MD
Professor and Chairman, Department of
Thoracic Surgery, Kyoto University Graduate
School of Medicine, Sakyo-ku, Kyoto, Japan

FEDERICO DAVINI, MD
Doctor, Thoracic Surgery, Cardiac and Thoracic
Department; Cardiothoracic and Vascular
Department, University of Pisa, Pisa, Italy

ANGELINA DE BENEDETTO, MD
Medical Oncology Division, Sapienza–
University of Rome, Rome, Italy

MAURIZIO DEL MONTE, MD
Department of Radiological Sciences, La
Sapienza University, Policlinico Umberto I,
Rome, Italy

JEAN DESLAURIERS, MD
Department of Thoracic Surgery, Institut
Universitaire de Cardiologie et de Pneumologie
de Québec (IUCPQ), Quebec City, Quebec,
Canada

FRANCESCO FAZI, PhD
Researcher, Department of Medico-Surgical
Sciences and Biotechnologies, Sapienza–
University of Rome, Latina, Italy

GIULIA FONTEMAGGI, PhD
Researcher, Translational Oncogenomics Unit,
Regina Elena Cancer Institute, Rome, Italy

FRANCESCO FRAIOLI, MD
Department of Radiological Sciences, La
Sapienza University, Policlinico Umberto I,
Rome, Italy

ÉRIC FRÉCHETTE, MD
Department of Thoracic Surgery, Institut
Universitaire de Cardiologie et de Pneumologie
de Québec (IUCPQ), Quebec City,
Quebec, Canada

JAROSŁAW KUŹDŻAŁ, MD, PhD, FETCS
Department of Thoracic Surgery, John Paul II
Hospital, Jagiellonian University, Cracow, Poland

FRANCA M.A. MELFI, MD
Doctor, Thoracic Surgery, Cardiac and Thoracic
Department; Cardiothoracic and Vascular
Department, University of Pisa, Pisa, Italy

MARIA LUISA MENNINI, MD
Department of Radiological Sciences,
La Sapienza University, Policlinico Umberto I,
Rome, Italy

BRYAN F. MEYERS, MD, MPH
Professor of Surgery, Division of
Cardiothoracic Surgery, Department of
Surgery, Washington University School of
Medicine, St. Louis, Missouri

DOUGLAS J. MINNICH, MD
Assistant Professor, Division of Cardiothoracic
Surgery, University of Alabama at Birmingham,
Birmingham, Alabama

ALFREDO MUSSI, MD
Cardiothoracic and Vascular Department,
University of Pisa; Professor of Thoracic
Surgery, Cardiac and Thoracic Department,
University of Pisa, Pisa, Italy

ANTONIO PASSARO, MD
Medical Oncology Division, Sapienza–
University of Rome, Rome, Italy

RAMÓN RAMI-PORTA, MD, PhD, FETCS
Attending Thoracic Surgeon, Thoracic Surgery
Service, Hospital Universitari Mutua Terrassa,
University of Barcelona, Terrassa,
Barcelona, Spain

ERINO A. RENDINA, MD
Professor and Chief, Department of Thoracic
Surgery, Sant'Andrea Hospital, University
La Sapienza, Rome, Italy

ARTUR SZLUBOWSKI, MD, PhD
Endoscopy Unit, John Paul II Hospital,
Cracow, Poland

PATRIZIA TRENTA, MD
Medical Oncology Division, Sapienza–
University of Rome, Rome, Italy

FEDERICO VENUTA, MD
Professor, Department of Thoracic Surgery,
Policlinico Umberto I; Fondazione Lorillard
Spencer-Cenci, University La Sapienza,
Rome, Italy

MARCIN ZIELIŃSKI, MD, PhD
Department of Thoracic Surgery, Pulmonary
Hospital, Zakopane, Poland

Contents

extended mediastinal lymphadenectomy (TEMLA). Both techniques enable the removal of the mediastinal nodes with the surrounding fatty tissue. VAMLA and TEMLA have very high diagnostic yield and can be combined with minimally invasive video-assisted lobectomy.

The Role of Lymphadenectomy in Lung Cancer Surgery

Antonio D'Andrilli, Federico Venuta, and Erino A. Rendina

Adequate lymphadenectomy represents a fundamental procedure in lung cancer surgery for accurate staging and potential survival benefit. Various techniques are used in current surgical practice for the intraoperative lymph node removal associated with pulmonary resection, without definitive indications concerning the preferable option. Different studies in the last decades have compared complete mediastinal lymph node dissection with lymph node sampling regarding their effect on long-term survival, recurrence rate, accuracy of pathologic staging, and surgical morbidity. Literature data and technical aspects of lymph node dissection are reported and discussed in this article.

The Impact of Complete Lymph Node Dissection for Lung Cancer on the Postoperative Course

Hiroshi Date

The role of lymph node dissection (LND) for non–small cell lung cancers (NSCLCs) remains controversial. LND adds little morbidity to a pulmonary resection for NSCLC, although it requires an additional 15 to 20 minutes of operative time. Four prospective randomized trials have been performed to compare lymph node sampling and LND; 3 trials showed no difference in survival and 1 showed survival benefit of LND. It is recommended that all patients with resectable NSCLC undergo LND because the procedure provides patients with the most accurate staging and the opportunity for effective adjuvant therapy.

The Impact of Chemotherapy on the Lymphatic System in Thoracic Oncology

Antonio Passaro, Patrizia Trenta, Davide Conte, Giuseppe Campennì, Angelina De Benedetto, and Enrico Cortesi

Non-small-cell lung cancer remains the leading cause of cancer-related mortality in the United States and Europe. Most patients are diagnosed with metastatic disease for which chemotherapy remains the cornerstone of treatment. In non-metastatic disease, surgery is the most potentially curative therapeutic option, but its outcome is still poor, in particular for patients with lymph node involvement. Therefore, several randomized adjuvant/neoadjuvant trials using chemotherapy and/or radiotherapy investigated the possibility of increasing the overall survival of patients with surgically treated lung cancer. The findings are reviewed in this article.

Index

Thoracic Surgery Clinics

READ THE CLINICS ONLINE!

Access your subscription at:
www.theclinics.com

Preface
The Lymphatic System in Thoracic Oncology

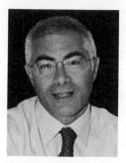 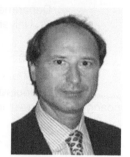

Federico Venuta, MD   Erino A. Rendina, MD
Guest Editors

This issue of *Thoracic Surgery Clinics* is dedicated to the lymphatic system in thoracic oncology. Scientific knowledge and technical options in this field of thoracic pathology have shown a significant improvement in recent years thanks to the joint efforts of surgeons, oncologists, radiologists, interventional pulmonologists, and pathologists.

Advances in technology and active clinical research in the last decades have contributed to increase the diagnostic accuracy and to modify the therapeutic approach when considering the lymphatic involvement in thoracic tumors. In particular, the introduction and progressive affirmation of some innovative diagnostic tools such as positron emission tomography and ultrasound-guided endoscopic procedures (EBUS, EUS) have partially modified the modern diagnostic approach to chest tumors. These techniques have made it possible to reduce the invasiveness of mediastinal staging and to extend the possibility of preoperative cytological or histologic sampling to lymph node stations that are not reachable by conventional surgical approaches (mediastinoscopy, anterior mediastinotomy, thoracoscopy).

In addition, a number of technical innovations have been introduced in thoracic surgery over time for the accomplishment of mediastinal lymph node dissection, with the aim of reducing the surgical trauma related to the standard approach through thoracotomy. These include thoracoscopic and robotic techniques and even the more recently proposed transcervical approach for extended mediastinal dissection Clinical investigation in this setting has also included the evaluation of alternative strategies such as the sentinel lymph node technique, which is actually the current surgical approach for lymph node exeresis in other extrathoracic tumors, to assess its potential benefit in lung cancer surgery.

Also, refinements in techniques and standardization of procedures in histopathological analysis have increased sensitivity significantly in the assessment of lymph node involvement by reducing the rate of undetected micrometastases. Moreover, recent applications of molecular biology

Thorac Surg Clin 22 (2012) ix–x
doi:10.1016/j.thorsurg.2012.02.001

in this field, including analysis of micro-RNA expression, are opening new perspectives in the definition of tumor biological behavior that could influence clinical practice in the near future.

All of the above-mentioned aspects are reported extensively and discussed in this issue. The scientific topics have been reviewed by a group of experts including all the specialities involved in the diagnosis and cure of oncologic chest diseases.

We would like to thank all the authors who have participated in this project. We are convinced that their outstanding contribution will provide readers with a complete overview of this interesting and complex topic.

Federico Venuta, MD
Department of Thoracic Surgery
University of Rome Sapienza
Policlinico Umberto I
V.le del Policlinico 155, Rome 00161, Italy

Erino A. Rendina, MD
Department of Thoracic Surgery
University of Rome Sapienza
Ospedale S.Andrea
V.le di Grottarossa 10035, Rome 161, Italy

E-mail addresses:
Federico.Venuta@uniroma1.it (F. Venuta)
erinoangelo.rendina@uniroma1.it (E.A. Rendina)

Anatomy and Physiology of the Thoracic Lymphatic System

Matias Losano Brotons, MD, Ciprian Bolca, MD, Éric Fréchette, MD, Jean Deslauriers, MD*

KEYWORDS

- Lymphatics of the thorax • Thoracic anatomy
- Anatomy of lymph nodes

Thoracic lymphatics play a significant role in the immune system of intrathoracic organs such as the lungs, pleura, esophagus, and mediastinum. Its network of lymphatic vessels carries interstitial fluid from the lungs, chyle from the digestive system, and white blood cells and other immune components. Thoracic lymphatics include the thymus and bone marrow, which are, with the spleen and digestive system lymphoid tissues, organs dedicated to lymphocyte production and circulation. Ultimately, thoracic lymphatics are related to a variety of pathologic processes that thoracic surgeons are asked to manage on a daily basis.

Of outmost importance is the role of this system in oncology where the lymphatic drainage of intrathoracic organs has now become a major point of interest for both thoracic surgeons and oncologists. Tumor staging, prognosis, and treatment are, for instance, largely dependent on the level of lymph node involvement. Similarly, operations done for intrathoracic malignancies generally include en bloc resection of local and regional draining lymph nodes because available data suggest that it may be associated with better outcomes.

This article is a review of the thoracic lymphatic system pertinent to thoracic surgeons, with a focus on embryologic, anatomic, and physiologic information needed to appreciate its significance in cancer management.

GENERALITIES ON THORACIC LYMPHATICS

The embryologic origin of the lymphatic system parallels that of the blood vasculature[1,2] as endothelial and hematopoietic cells arise from the hemangioblast, which is the common mesodermal-derived progenitor cell. This cell is the only cell able to generate all components of the vascular system, even if multiple molecular signals are necessary to allow the proper differentiation of lymphatic endothelial cells into a functional lymphatic system (**Fig. 1**).[3] Although thoracic lymphatics derive from a venous precursor,[4–7] they usually do not communicate with the venous system except where the left thoracic duct and right thoracic duct join the left and right venous jugular-subclavian confluences, respectively.[8,9] The lymphatic system of the heart and mediastinum is established at the end of embryonic life and is complete by early postfetal life,[10] whereas bronchopulmonary lymph nodes fully develop during the years after birth.

Along their course within the lung or mediastinum, all lymphatic collectors flow into lymph nodes, which are an important part of the lymphatic

Conflicts of interest: None.
Department of Thoracic Surgery, Institut Universitaire de Cardiologie et de Pneumologie de Québec (IUCPQ), 2725 Chemin Sainte-Foy, Quebec City, Quebec G1V 4G5, Canada
* Corresponding author.
E-mail address: jean.deslauriers@chg.ulaval.ca

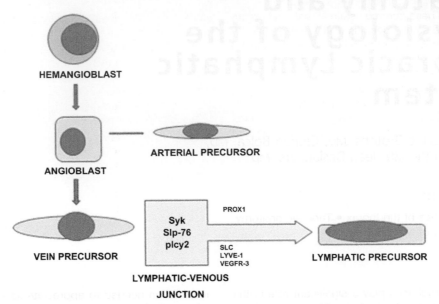

Fig. 1. Embryologic origin of the lymphatic system. Note that the hemangioblast is the common precursor of all components of the vascular system, including the lymphatic vessels. The lymphatic differentiation comes from a venous precursor, and some spatially located receptors are necessary for the formation of lymphatic-venous connections. LYVE-1, lymphatic vessel hyaluronan receptor 1; PROX1, prospero-related homeo box-1; SLC, secondary lymphoid chemokine; Slp-76 and plcy2, signaling adaptor proteins; Syk, spleen tyrosine kinase; VEGFR-3, vessel endothelial growth factor 3.

system. Those structures form pathways called lymph node chains, which eventually drain into the systemic circulation either through direct connections at the level of the cervical venous confluence or indirectly via the thoracic duct.

The number, size, and location of the collecting channels and lymph nodes are variable among individuals and even within the same individual, and such variability must be taken into account while doing surgery for thoracic malignancies. Lymphatics from the lungs, for instance, usually drain in the ipsilateral mediastinal nodes, but they will, on occasion, drain in the contralateral mediastinum after crossing over at the level of the lower trachea.[11]

LYMPHATIC SYSTEM OF THORACIC ORGANS AND STRUCTURES
Chest Wall

The anterior part of the intercostal space drains into parasternal nodes located at the anterior end of the intercostal spaces along each internal mammary artery, whereas their efferents unite with those of the tracheobronchial and brachiocephalic nodes. The posterior part of the intercostal space drains into the intercostal nodes located near the heads and necks of the ribs. Efferents of the lower 4 to 7 spaces unite to form a common trunk that descends to the intra-abdominal cisterna chyli or

drains directly at the origin of the thoracic duct. Efferents of the left upper spaces end in the thoracic duct, whereas those of the right upper spaces end in one of the right lymphatic trunks.

The intercostal lymphatic vessels draining the inner intercostal layer and parietal pleura consist of a single trunk in each space, and these trunks run forward in the subpleural tissues. The trunks of the upper 6 spaces open separately in the internal mammary nodes, whereas those of the lower spaces unite to form a single trunk that terminates in the lowest part of the internal mammary nodal chain.[12,13]

Pleura and Pleural Spaces

The pleural space is on the boundary of 2 lymphatic systems, both of which play a significant role in fluid resorption and removal of foreign particles, cells, and proteins from that space.

In the subpleural space of the visceral pleura, large lymphatic capillaries form a meshed network that drains into the pulmonary lymphatic system and is called the superficial lymphatic plexus of the lung. These capillaries are more abundant over the lower lobes and are connected to the deep pulmonary plexus located in the interlobular and peribronchial spaces.

The lymphatic drainage of the parietal pleura is more elaborate, with direct communications between the pleural space and the parietal lymphatic channels. These communications, called stomata (**Box 1**), are small openings (8–10 μm) formed by discontinuities in the mesothelium of the parietal pleura.[14] They are round or oval, and their density predominates over the lower portions of the mediastinal, diaphragmatic, and costal pleura. The stomata are the major route for pleural fluid resorption as well as for the removal of foreign particles and cells.[15,16] They have endoluminal valves and drain into a network of submesothelial lacunae. Over the costal pleura, the collecting vessels run parallel to the ribs to reach the internal mammary nodal chain anteriorly and the intercostal nodal chain posteriorly. At the level of the diaphragm, the drainage is to the retrosternal, mediastinal, and celiac nodes. These transdiaphragmatic anastomoses allow for the passage of fluid and foreign particles from the peritoneal cavity into the pleural space.

Lungs

Among human organs, the lungs have, by far, the largest exposed surface to an environment containing particulates, toxic matters, bacteria, and viruses; in addition, it is constantly irrigated by large amounts of blood arising from a highly specialized vascular system. Under such circumstances, the lungs require an efficient lymphatic system not only able to keep them dry even in the event of massive fluid challenges but also able to clear inert and toxic matters that may penetrate the epithelium.[17]

Even though there are some older descriptions of pulmonary lymphatics, Henri Rouvière,[18] a French anatomist, is generally credited with the first comprehensive documentation of the lymphatic system of the lungs. Through selective injection of lymph vessels in human autopsy specimens, Rouvière accurately described the lymphatic drainage of each pulmonary lobe and even conceptualized the idea of specific lymph node involvement based on the anatomic origin of lung tumors or of tuberculous lesions. In the 1950s, additional and important contributions were those of Borrie[19] and Nohl.[20] More recently, Marc Riquet and others[11,21,22] revisited those earlier descriptions through carefully done studies on human cadavers and provided new and pertinent information regarding the lymphatic spread of lung cancer to the mediastinum.

The lungs have a highly developed lymphatic network (**Box 2**) consisting of a subpleural superficial plexus located within the connective tissues of the visceral pleura and a deep peribronchovascular plexus located in the connective tissues surrounding the airways, pulmonary arteries, and veins. The subpleural lymphatics run under the surface of the lung, predominantly over the lower lobes, toward the hilum where they anastomose with the lymphatics of the deep plexus.[23] It is generally accepted that the superficial plexus takes up the lymph from the visceral pleura and adjoining layer of subpleural tissues, whereas the remaining lung is drained by the peribronchovascular deep plexus. On occasion, subpleural lymphatic collectors can connect directly in the mediastinum,[22] thus explaining the presence of skipped metastasis in about 10% to 15% of patients with primary lung cancer.

The fusion of lymphatic capillaries of the deep plexus forms a network of lymphatic collecting vessels called collectors, which contain unidirectional valves and smooth muscle within their walls. These collecting vessels are not as rigid as systemic blood vessels and their diameter varies irrespective of their course; indeed, their size can double just a few millimeters upstream or downstream. Larger lymphatic collectors have 3 well-defined layers that includes an intima with a lymphatic endothelium and a continuous basal membrane, a media that has the role of active propulsion through a valvelike system, also called second valve system, and an adventitia made up mainly of collagen and fibroblast bundles.[24] Because of these nearly all bicuspid regularly

---

Box 1
Characteristics of pleural stomata

- Small openings (8–10 μm) in mesothelium of parietal pleura

- Round or oval

- Have endoluminal valves

- Predominate over the lower parietal pleura (costal, diaphragmatic)

- Major route for pleural fluid resorption

- Not present in visceral pleura

Box 2
Lymphatic plexuses of the lung

Plexus	Location
Superficial	Connective tissues under visceral pleura
Deep	Connective tissues surrounding airways, pulmonary arteries and veins

distributed 1-way valves (every 2–10 mm),[25,26] lymph flow is in the direction of the hilum.

Scattered lymphocytes and plasma cells are also found in the wall of the tracheobronchial tree, creating lymphoid nodules that are mainly covered with nonciliated lymphoepithelium. These are known as bronchus-associated lymphoid tissue, and they have a morphologic resemblance to the intestinal Peyer patches.[27]

Earlier studies[18–20] performed on tumors located in various parts of the lungs showed that lymphatic drainage and nodal pathways are largely dependent on the lobar origin of the tumor. Malignant lesions of the right upper lobe, for instance, drain preferentially to the right hilum and then to the right paratracheal lymph node chain (**Box 3**). A cluster of lymph nodes called the lymphatic pulmonary sump or sump of Borrie[19,20] is always present below the origin of the upper lobe bronchus on both the left (**Fig. 2**A) and right side (see **Fig. 2**B). Because these sump nodes receive lymph flow from all lobes, the clinical implication is that one may have to consider pneumonectomy (vs lobectomy) if these nodes contain metastatic tumor. The right middle and lower lobes usually drain into the subcarinal nodes and secondarily into the right paratracheal lymph node chain. In about one-third of cases, tumors located in the left upper lobe will have an alternate pathway to subaortic, periaortic, and anterior mediastinal nodes, whereas left lower lobe tumors drain into the subcarinal and left tracheobronchial chain.

Because of the multiple connections that exist between lymphatic channels, mediastinal metastases may occur in any of the mediastinal lymph nodes regardless of the anatomic origin of the tumor. Hilar nodes can sometimes be bypassed, and mediastinal metastases occur without hilar involvement (skipped metastases), a phenomenon more often encountered in tumors located in upper lobes. Bronchial lymphatics from both lungs have a tendency to remain ipsilateral, but they may sometimes connect with the contralateral mediastinum after crossing over, usually at the level of the lower trachea or subcarinal space.[11]

Pericardium and Heart

The pericardium consists of 2 layers of mesothelial cells with lamellar connective tissue between them. Lymphatic stomata are only found in the inner layer where they have a scattered distribution. Pericardial stomata connect with submesothelial lymphatic vessels, and the drainage is eventually directed toward the tracheobronchial nodes (lateral pericardium) and paraesophageal nodes (posterior pericardium). The lymphatic vessels of the anterior pericardium most often pass along the phrenic nerves to terminate in the nodes of the anterior mediastinum.[28] These anatomic observations offer new insights into the mediastinal drainage of lung tumors invading the pericardium[29] that are generally considered to have a worse prognosis even after complete resection.

The lymphatic system of the heart consists of 3 plexuses (**Box 4**).[30] The endocardial plexus, which is a network of small lymphatic capillaries located below the basal membrane of the endocardium, has an enormous potential for dilatation, and drains into a deeper plexus called the myocardial plexus that has a drainage pattern that generally follows the coronary blood vessels toward the epicardium. The third plexus, called the epicardial plexus, collects effluents from the subendocardial and myocardial plexuses, and it is a loosely interconnected network located in the subepicardial connective tissues. It reaches the collector lymphatic channels over the surface of the heart and eventually coalesces into cardiac lymphatic trunks.

The left main cardiac lymphatic trunk collects lymph from a left branch (anterior surface of the left ventricle) and a right branch (posterior surface of the left ventricle and left atrium), which unite under the left atrial appendage. It runs behind and along the left main pulmonary artery and eventually passes to the left of the aortic root and ascending aorta toward the aortic arch. The right main cardiac lymphatic trunk, which collects lymph from the right ventricle and right atrium, is located over the posterior surface of the heart. It runs along the interventricular groove toward the base of heart and, similar to the course of the right coronary artery, curves toward the anterior surface of the right ventricle in the direction of the right atrial appendage and ascending aorta. From there,

---

Box 3
Usual lymphatic drainage of each lobe of the lung

Right lung

Upper lobe: superior mediastinum

Middle lobe: superior or posteroinferior mediastinum

Lower lobe: inferior mediastinum

Left lung

Upper lobe: superior and anterior mediastinum

Lower lobe: inferior mediastinum

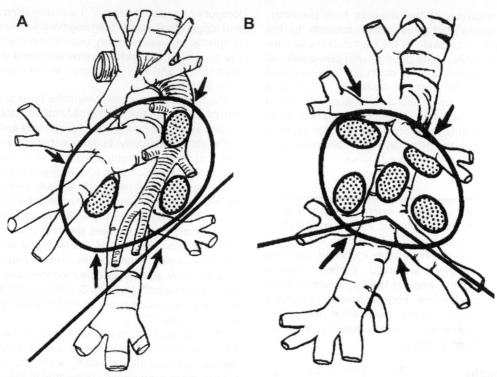

Fig. 2. (*A*) Left lymphatic sump that corresponds to a cluster of nodes located below the junction of the origins left upper and lower lobe bronchi and (*B*) right lymphatic sump that lies between the origin of the right upper lobe bronchus proximally and those of the middle lobe and superior segment of the lower lobe distally. The arrows indicate the direction of lymphatic drainage from each lobe to the sump area. (*Reprinted from* Nohl HC. An investigation into the lymphatic and vascular spread of carcinoma of the bronchus. Thorax 1956;11:172–85; with permission.)

the right main cardiac lymphatic trunk travels in the direction of the aortopulmonary window where it unites with the left trunk to reach the nodes located in that area.

Diaphragm

The lymphatic drainage of the diaphragm consists of 3 groups of lymph nodes (**Box 5**). The anterolateral portion of the diaphragm drains into nodes located at the lowest part of the internal mammary chain, adjacent to the xiphoid process. The middle or juxtaphrenic groups are located near the entrance point of the phrenic nerves, and they eventually drain into periesophageal, pulmonary ligament, and tracheobronchial nodes.[31] The posterior or retrocrural nodes usually drain inferiorly across the diaphragmatic crura to the para-aortic lymph nodes located around the celiac trunk and renal arteries. In some cases, the lymph from the diaphragm can drain directly into the thoracic duct without crossing any intervening nodes.

Box 4 Lymphatics of the heart	
Plexus	**Location**
Endocardial	Below the basal membrane of endocardium
Myocardial	Intramyocardial
Epicardial	Subepicardial connective tissues

Box 5 Lymphatics of the diaphragm	
Location	**Site of Drainage**
Anterolateral portion of diaphragm	Lowest part of internal mammary chain
Middle or juxtaphrenic	Periesophageal nodes, inferior pulmonary ligament nodes, tracheobronchial nodes
Posterior or retrocrural	Para-aortic nodes

The anatomy of the effluents from diaphragmatic nodes that drain either caudally to the abdomen or cranially to the tracheobronchial nodes may explain why patients with non–small cell lung cancer invading the diaphragm have a worse prognosis after surgical resection.[32–34] In one interesting review, Yokoi and colleagues[35] stated that primary lung tumors with diaphragmatic invasion, especially invasion of the muscle layer or deep tissues, are generally technically resectable but oncologically almost incurable.

Thymus

As a primary lymphatic organ, the thymus does not have afferent lymphatics. According to Safieddine and Keshavjee,[36] 3 groups of efferent lymphatic vessels have been identified, and they include superior lymphatic vessels draining directly into the internal jugular, innominate, or anterior mediastinal nodes; anterior lymphatic ducts draining into the parasternal nodes; and posterior lymphatic ducts draining into the tracheobronchial nodes.

Esophagus

The esophageal lymphatic drainage presents some special features as it crosses 3 anatomic regions (neck, thorax, and abdomen) and has a foregut embryologic origin.[37] It is mainly intramural and longitudinal, rather than segmental. There are lymphatic plexuses in every esophageal layer, but the lymphatic network is more abundant in the submucosa and less developed in the muscular layer (**Fig. 3**).

The dense submucosal lymphatic layer is uninterrupted and connects with the lymphatic submucosal layer of the hypopharynx proximally and that of the stomach distally. In general, the upper two-thirds of the esophagus drain cephalad and the lower third drains caudad toward the abdomen.

The submucosal lymphatic vessels penetrate, sometimes independently, the muscularis propria (either the outer or the inner layer) without any concomitant artery and vein, creating connections with lymphatic plexuses at this level and with the paraesophageal lymph nodes. This submucosal network may also have direct connections with the thoracic duct[38] (see **Fig. 3**), although the exact patterns and occurrences of these pathways are highly variable.[39–42]

Most cervical lymph nodes draining the esophagus are located near the recurrent laryngeal nerves and carotid sheaths, whereas, in the thorax, most such nodes are located in the region of the tracheobronchial bifurcation and pulmonary hilum. In the chest, these nodes drain both the esophagus and lung, and the direction of the

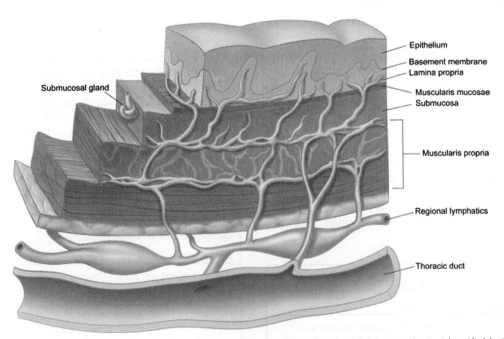

Epithelium

Basement membrane

Lamina propria

Muscularis mucosae

Submucosa

Muscularis propria

Regional lymphatics

Thoracic duct

Submucosal gland

Fig. 3. Intramural and regional lymphatics of the esophagus. Note that lymphatic vessels are identifiable in the mucosa, submucosa, and muscularis propria. Lymph can drain directly into the thoracic duct or relay through regional lymphatic and lymph nodes. (*Courtesy of* Cleveland Clinic and The Cleveland Clinic Foundation, with permission.)

lymph flow may be either cephalad or caudad.[39] Below the carina and pulmonary hilum, most lymph flow proceeds downstream, in the direction of the esophagogastric junction to the perigastric nodal groups including the celiac nodes.

LYMPHATIC COLLECTORS OF THE MEDIASTINUM

The lymphatic collectors of the mediastinum (**Box 6**) (**Fig. 4**) originate from the deep lymphatic channels of the lungs. Their drainage is generally ipsilateral, but anomalies can be encountered, usually on the left side, where lower lobe collectors may drain through the subcarinal lymphatic channels to right-sided mediastinal nodes in up to one-third of individuals.

In general, lymphatic collectors of the inferior mediastinum travel upstream within the inferior pulmonary ligaments and ascend toward the carina. Thus, tumors of the lower lobes have a tendency to spread to subcarinal nodes and from there continue on to either side of the trachea. On occasion, collectors from the inferior mediastinum travel downstream, traversing the diaphragm to terminate in the intra-abdominal periaortic nodes.[43–45]

Lymphatic collectors of the superior mediastinum are numerous, and most ascend along the lateral and anterior aspects of the trachea. On the right side (right pretracheal lymphatic collector), they terminate in the venous circulation through 1 or several arches,[46] whereas, on the left side (left pretracheal lymphatic collector), the collectors travel cephalad along the left recurrent nerve (lateral aspect of the trachea) to eventually terminate into the venous system at the left jugular-subclavian venous confluence. Because of these particularities, upper lobe tumors seldom metastasize to subcarinal nodes.

Additional and important lymphatic collectors of the superior mediastinum include a right posterior

lymphatic collector (tracheoesophageal collector), which ascends between the right lateral aspect of the trachea and lateral border of the esophagus and a group of left preaortic collectors, which are located in the anterior mediastinum and run upward along the aortic arch to terminate into the left jugular-subclavian confluence.[11]

NODAL CHAINS OF THE MEDIASTINUM

The lymphatic collectors and the nodes located along their course form pathways named lymph node chains. In the thorax, there are 3 main lymphatic pathways that include a posterior parietal chain ascending in the posterior mediastinum along the spine, an anterior parietal chain ascending along the internal mammary vessels, and a median visceral chain ascending along the tracheobronchial tree and phrenic nerves. There is also a diaphragmatic lymphatic network that drains the diaphragm and connects with all 3 main ascendant pathways. The thoracic duct is the main lymphatic vessel to which all lymphatic networks eventually drain.

The posterior parietal chain that ascends in the posterior mediastinum collects intercostal lymphatics draining the chest wall, the posterior parietal pleura, and the posterior part of the diaphragm. Over their course, there are lymph nodes located in the extrapleural fat adjacent to the heads of the ribs (posterior intercostal nodes). The drainage of this posterior network is essentially ascendant on both sides terminating in the thoracic duct or directly into the angle of Pirogoff. On occasion, this network drains inferiorly and in such cases involves the lymphatics located within the gastrohepatic ligament and celiac nodes.

The anterior thoracic chain that ascends along the internal mammary vessels drains the anterior chest wall, the anterior and lateral diaphragm, and the medial breast. The internal mammary nodes are found in the intercostal spaces along the sternum and are usually present from the fifth intercostal spaces to the clavicles. Like the posterior network, this chain can also drain inferiorly through the rectus abdominis muscle sheath to the subdiaphragmatic and subperitoneal plexuses and forward to the liver and retroperitoneal nodes. There are also connections between left and right anterior thoracic chains through intercostal channels.

The median visceral chain collects branches from the posterior paraesophageal chain, some from the anterior chain along the phrenic nerves and, most importantly, from the median tracheobronchial chain, which essentially drain the lungs.

Box 6 Lymphatic collectors of the mediastinum	
Site of Collector	**Site of Drainage**
Inferior mediastinum	Subcarinal nodes Intra-abdominal nodes
Superior mediastinum	Nodes located over anterolateral aspect of trachea
Anterior mediastinum	Left jugular-subclavian confluence

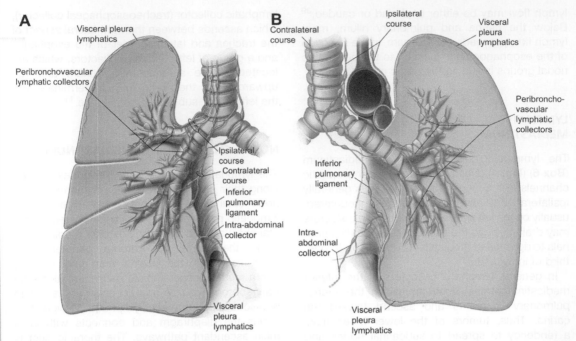

Fig. 4. (*A*) Visceral pleura lymphatics and peribronchial vascular lymphatic collectors of the right lung. (*B*) Visceral pleura lymphatics and peribronchial vascular lymphatic collectors of the left lung. (*Reprinted from* Riquet M. Bronchial arteries and lymphatic of the lung. Thorac Surg Clin 2007;17:627. Figure 6; p. 628. Figure 7; with permission.)

ANATOMIC DISTRIBUTION OF MEDIASTINAL NODES AND NODE CLASSIFICATION FOR LUNG CANCER

Although the anatomy of thoracic lymph nodes has been known for a long time, these nodes have recently been regrouped in nodal stations that are pertinent to surgeons operating on thoracic malignancies, mainly lung cancer (**Fig. 5**). Although this work was originally done in Japan by Naruke and colleagues,[47] it was modified in 1997 by Mountain and Dressler[48] to correlate basic anatomy with new imaging technologies such as computed tomographic scanning. In this regional classification, lymph nodes located within the lung (bronchopulmonary nodes) are classified as being in stations 11 to 14, nodes located in the hilum (hilar nodes) are included in station 10, and nodes from the mediastinum are classified as being in stations 1 to 9 depending on their location. The anatomic boundary between hilar and mediastinal nodes is the mediastinal pleura.

Nodes of the Posteroinferior Mediastinum (Stations 7, 8, 9)

Nodes of the posteroinferior mediastinum are largely paraesophageal (station 8) and subcarinal (station 7). Nodes of the inferior pulmonary ligament (station 9) are few (2–3), and they lie in close

proximity to the inferior pulmonary vein. These nodes may connect with the para-aortic nodes in the abdomen, a consideration that is most important in cases of lower thoracic esophageal carcinomas. Lymph nodes of the tracheal bifurcation (station 7) are variable in number and size, and they are arranged in clusters, one being located anteriorly and a second one more posteriorly and extending laterally to the main bronchi. The nodes located anteriorly are easily accessed by mediastinoscopy, but those located posteriorly can only be accessed by ultrasound techniques (endoscopic ultrasonography, endobronchial ultrasonography) or video-thoracoscopy. The paraesophageal nodes (station 8) are mostly involved with the esophageal lymph drainage.

Nodes of the Superior Mediastinum (Stations 1, 2, 4)

These nodes constitute the most important group of mediastinal nodes. The tracheobronchial nodes (station 4) are located in the angle between the trachea and corresponding main bronchus. On the right side, they are situated medial to the arch of the azygos vein and above the right pulmonary artery, whereas, on the left, they lie in the concavity of the aortic arch. The superior paratracheal nodes (station 2) are located higher up along the anterolateral wall of the trachea

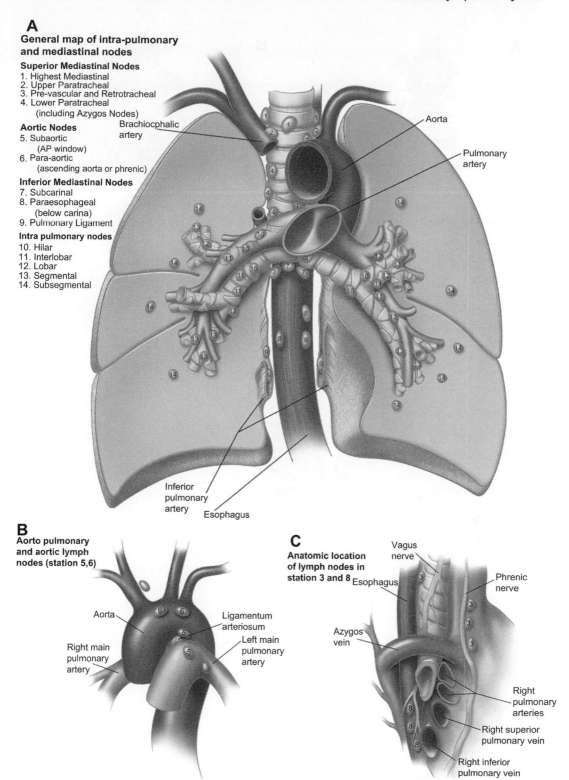

A

General map of intra-pulmonary and mediastinal nodes

Superior Mediastinal Nodes
1. Highest Mediastinal
2. Upper Paratracheal
3. Pre-vascular and Retrotracheal
4. Lower Paratracheal
   (including Azygos Nodes)

Aortic Nodes
5. Subaortic
   (AP window)
6. Para-aortic
   (ascending aorta or phrenic)

Inferior Mediastinal Nodes
7. Subcarinal
8. Paraesophageal
   (below carina)
9. Pulmonary Ligament

Intra pulmonary nodes
10. Hilar
11. Interlobar
12. Lobar
13. Segmental
14. Subsegmental

Brachiocephalic artery

Aorta

Pulmonary artery

Inferior pulmonary artery

Esophagus

B

Aorto pulmonary and aortic lymph nodes (station 5,6)

Aorta

Right main pulmonary artery

Ligamentum arteriosum

Left main pulmonary artery

C

Anatomic location of lymph nodes in station 3 and 8

Vagus nerve

Esophagus

Phrenic nerve

Azygos vein

Right pulmonary arteries

Right superior pulmonary vein

Right inferior pulmonary vein

Fig. 5. Regional nodal classification for lung cancer staging. (*A*) Lymph nodes of the lung and posteroinferior and superior mediastinum. (*B*) Aortic nodes. (*C*) Right prevascular and retrotracheal nodes. (*From* Riquet M. Bronchial arteries and lymphatic of the lung. Thorac Surg 2007;17:619–38, p. 634, Figure 11, with permission; data from Mountain CF, Dresler CM. Regional lymph node classification for lung cancer staging. Chest 1997;111:1718–23.)

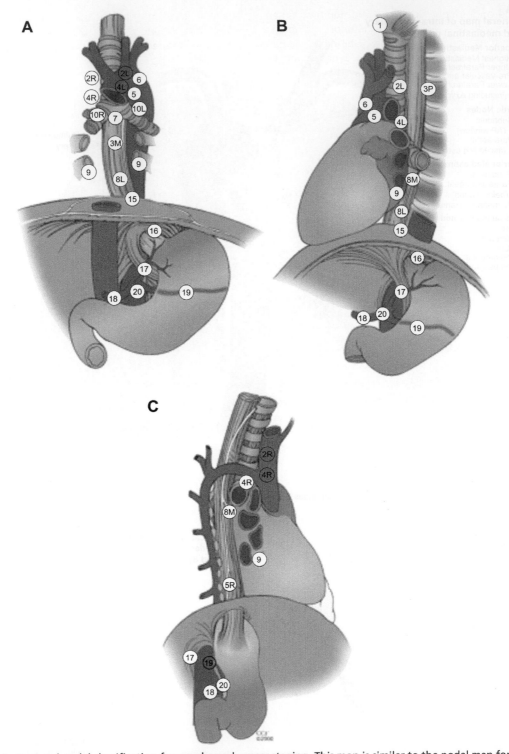

Fig. 6. Regional nodal classification for esophageal cancer staging. This map is similar to the nodal map for lung cancer, but station 8 is subdivided into 8M (middle paraesophageal) and 8L (lower paraesophageal). Specific stations include 15 (diaphragmatic), 16 (paracardial), 17 (left gastric), 18 (common hepatic), 19 (splenic), and 20 (celiac). *A*, anterior view; *B*, left lateral view; *C*, right lateral view. (*Courtesy of* Thomas W. Rice. *From* Rice TW. Diagnosis and staging of esophageal cancer. In: Patterson GA, Pearson FG, Cooper JD, et al, editors. Pearson's thoracic and esophageal surgery. vol. 2. Esophageal, Philadelphia: Churchill Livingstone, Elsevier Inc., 2008; with permission.)

Those on the right side are more numerous than on the left side, and they lie inferior and to the right of the innominate artery. Still higher lymph nodes are located in station 1 where they lie above a horizontal line at the upper rim of the innominate artery. These nodes form the link between tracheobronchial nodes and inferior deep cervical nodes.

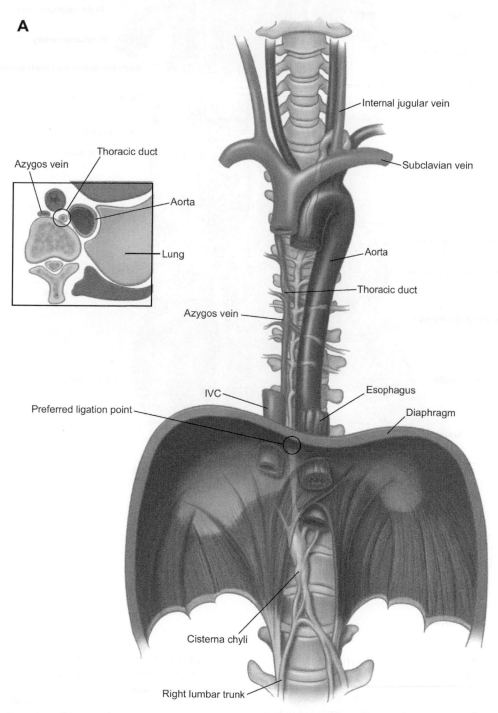

A

Azygos vein

Thoracic duct

Aorta

Lung

Internal jugular vein

Subclavian vein

Aorta

Thoracic duct

Azygos vein

IVC

Esophagus

Diaphragm

Preferred ligation point

Cisterna chyli

Right lumbar trunk

Fig. 7. Anatomy of the thoracic duct (*A*) Anterior view showing the preferred point of thoracic duct mass ligation in the surgical treatment of chylothorax. (*B*) Posterior view of the duct and its tributaries. (*From* Hematti H, Mehran RJ. Anatomy of the thoracic duct. Thorac Surg Clin 2011;21:232, 234; with permission.)

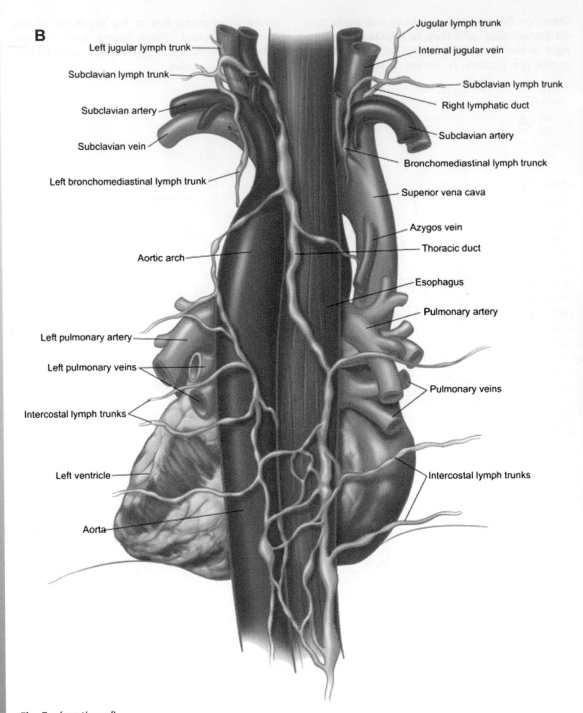

B

Left jugular lymph trunk

Subclavian lymph trunk

Subclavian artery

Subclavian vein

Left bronchomediastinal lymph trunk

Aortic arch

Left pulmonary artery

Left pulmonary veins

Intercostal lymph trunks

Left ventricle

Aorta

Jugular lymph trunk

Internal jugular vein

Subclavian lymph trunk

Right lymphatic duct

Subclavian artery

Bronchomediastinal lymph trunk

Superior vena cava

Azygos vein

Thoracic duct

Esophagus

Pulmonary artery

Pulmonary veins

Intercostal lymph trunks

Fig. 7. (continued)

Nodes of the Anterior Mediastinum (Stations 5, 6)

These nodes are numerous, and they overlie the upper portion of the pericardium. Nodes of station 5 are located in the aortopulmonary window in close proximity to the origin of the left pulmonary artery and the ligamentum arteriosum, whereas nodes of station 6 are deeply embedded between the origins of the left carotid and left subclavian arteries. These nodes, which are particularly important in the lymphatic drainage of the left upper lobe, lie underneath the mediastinal pleura between the phrenic and vagus nerves.

ANATOMIC DISTRIBUTION OF THE MEDIASTINAL NODES AND NODES CLASSIFICATION FOR ESOPHAGEAL CANCER

This nodal map uses the previously described nodal stations for lung cancer with specific modifications for esophageal cancer (**Fig. 6**), which includes subdividing station 8 into middle and lower paraesophageal nodes and the addition of stations 15 to 20.

ANATOMY AND PHYSIOLOGY OF THE THORACIC DUCT

The thoracic duct is the main collecting vessel of the lymphatic system. It is approximately 45 cm in length and 2 to 5 mm in diameter. The volume of flow through the thoracic duct is between 60 and 190 mL/h,[49] and, like all larger lymph collectors, it has a media made of smooth muscle fibers that contract periodically to aid lymph flow movement and a valve system that prevents retrograde flow. Although the number of such valves is variable, there is one consistent valve at the venous confluence that protects the thoracic duct against the reflux of blood.

The thoracic duct extends from L2 to the base of the neck (**Fig. 7**), and it collects lymph from the entire body except from the right side of the head and neck, right hemithorax, and right upper extremity. The thoracic duct originates (abdominal part) from the cranial portion of the cisterna chyli, which is a dilated lymph sac located behind the right diaphragmatic crus over the surface of L2. It then passes through the aortic hiatus of the diaphragm (T10) with the aorta to its left and the azygos vein (thoracic part) to its right (see **Fig. 7**A). It then ascends the posterior mediastinum up to the level of T5, where it inclines to the left to enter the superior mediastinum and ascend to the left side of the esophagus toward the thoracic inlet. At that level (cervical part), the duct arches behind the innominate vein (about 4 cm above the clavicle), and it usually ends by opening into the junction of the left subclavian and internal jugular vein.

Variability in the anatomy of the thoracic duct is the rule with 40% to 60% of individuals having anomalous venous connections with the azygos, intercostal, and lumbar veins and as much as 25% to 30% of individuals having multiple ducts at the diaphragmatic level. There is also extreme variability in the termination of the thoracic duct at the cervical venous confluence.[50–52]

Several tributaries join the thoracic duct along its course, and these include descending paired posterior intercostal collectors that drain the 6 or 7 lower intercostal spaces, ascending upper intercostal trunks, and direct duct tributaries draining lymph from thoracic organs without any intervening lymph nodes.[53]

The right thoracic (lymphatic) duct is small (2 cm in length), and it typically forms from the union of 3 lymphatic trunks: the right jugular, the right subclavian, and the right bronchomediastinal trunks. In most cases, the duct is closely related to the anterior scalene muscle and empties into the junction of the right subclavian and right internal jugular veins.

SUMMARY

The thoracic lymphatic system is one of the most complex and poorly understood systems of the human body, and much is still to be learned, especially in lymphatic physiology. Knowledge of the normal anatomy of this system as well as of its variations is nevertheless important for thoracic surgeons investigating and treating patients with lung or esophageal neoplasms.

REFERENCES

1. Oliver G, Detmar M. The rediscovery of the lymphatic system: old and new insights into the development and biological function of the lymphatic vasculature. Genes Dev 2002;16:773–83.
2. Tammela T, Alitalo K. Lymphangiogenesis: molecular mechanisms and future promise. Cell 2010; 140(4):460–76.
3. Jain RK, Padera TP. Lymphatics make the break. Science 2003;299:209–10.
4. Sarin F. The lymphatic system in human embryos with a consideration of the morphology of the system as a whole. Am J Anat 1909;IX(1):43–91.
5. Srinivasan RS, Dillard ME, Lagutin OV, et al. Lineage tracing demonstrates the venous origin of the mammalian lymphatic vasculature. Genes Dev 2007;21(19):2422–32.
6. Harvey N, Oliver G. Choose your fate: artery, vein or lymphatic vessel? Curr Opin Genet Dev 2004;14(5): 499–505.
7. Hong Y, Detmar M. Prox1, master regulator of the lymphatic vasculature phenotype. Cell Tissue Res 2003;314(1):85–92.
8. Butler M, Isogai S, Weinstein B. Lymphatic development. Birth Defects Res C Embryo Today 2009; 87(3):222–31.
9. Abtahian F, Guerriero A, Sebzda E, et al. Regulation of blood and lymphatic vascular separation by signaling proteins SLP-76 and Syk. Science 2003; 299(5604):247–51.
10. Riquet M, Brière J, Dupont P, et al. The embryonic and early fetal development of the lymphatics of

the heart and lungs in humans. Surg Radiol Anat 1993;15:369–70.

11. Riquet M. Bronchial arteries and lymphatics of the lung. Thorac Surg Clin 2007;17:619–38.

12. Rendina EA, Ciccone AM. The intercostal space. Thorac Surg Clin 2007;17:491–501.

13. Gray H. Gray's anatomy: the anatomical basis of clinical practice. Philadelphia: Elsevier; 2005. p. 966. Chapter 6.

14. Sevin M, Light RW. Anatomy of the pleura. Thorac Surg Clin 2011;21:173–5.

15. Wang NS. The preformed stomas connecting the pleural cavity and the lymphatics in the parietal pleura. Am Rev Respir Dis 1975;111: 12–20.

16. Li J. Ultrastructural study on the pleural stomata in human. Funct Dev Morphol 1993;3:277–80.

17. Schaufnagel DE. Lung lymphatic anatomy and correlates. Pathophysiology 2010;17:337–43.

18. Rouvière H. Les vaisseaux lymphatiques des poumons et les ganglions viscéraux intrathoraciques. Ann Anat Pathol 1929;65:113–58 [in French].

19. Borrie J. Primary carcinoma of the bronchus: prognosis following surgical resection. Ann R Coll Surg Engl 1950;10:165–86.

20. Nohl HC. An investigation into the lymphatic and vascular spread of carcinoma of the bronchus. Thorax 1956;11:172–85.

21. Riquet M. Anatomic basis of lymphatic spread from carcinoma of the lung to the mediastinum. Surgical and prognostic implications. Surg Radiol Anat 1993;15:271–7.

22. Riquet M, Hidden G, Debesse B. Direct lymphatic drainage of lung segments to the mediastinal nodes. Anatomical study on 200 adults. J Thorac Cardiovasc Surg 1989;97:623–32.

23. Lauweryns JM, Baert JH. Alveolar clearance and the role of the pulmonary lymphatics. Am Rev Respir Dis 1977;115:625–83.

24. Schmid-Schönbein GW. The second valve system in lymphatics. Lymphat Res Biol 2003;1:25–9 [discussion: 29–31].

25. Drake RE, Weiss D, Gabel JC. Active lymphatic pumping and sheep lung lymph flow. J Appl Physiol 1991;71:99–103.

26. Zawieja DC. Contractile physiology of lymphatics. Lymphat Res Biol 2009;7:87–96.

27. Murray JF, editor. The normal lung: the basis for diagnosis and treatment of pulmonary disease. 2nd edition. Philadelphia: WB Saunders Co; 2006. Chapter 3. p. 61–82.

28. Eliskoua M, Eliska O, Miller AJ. The lymphatic drainage of the parietal pericardium in man. Lymphology 1995; 28:208–17.

29. Riquet M, Le Pimbec-Barthes F, Hidden G. Lymphatic drainage of the pericardium to the mediastinal lymph nodes. Surg Radiol Anat 2001;23:317–9.

30. Schmid-Schönbein GW. Microlymphatics and lymph flow. Physiol Rev 1990;70:987–1027.

31. Souilamas R, Hidden G, Riquet M. Mediastinal efferents from the diaphragm. Surg Radiol Anat 2001;23: 159–62.

32. Weksler B, Bains M, Burt M, et al. Resection of lung cancer involving the diaphragm. J Thorac Cardiovasc Surg 1977;114:500–1.

33. Rocco G, Rendina EA, Meroni A, et al. Prognostic factors after surgical treatment of lung cancer involving the diaphragm. Ann Thorac Surg 1999;68:2065–8.

34. Riquet M, Porte H, Chapelier A, et al. Resection of lung cancer involving the diaphragm. J Thorac Cardiovasc Surg 2000;120:417–8.

35. Yokoi K, Tsuchiya R, Mori T, et al. Results of surgical treatment of lung cancer invading the diaphragm. J Thorac Cardiovasc Surg 2000;120:799–805.

36. Safieddine N, Keshavjee S. Anatomy of the thymus gland. Thorac Surg Clin 2011;21:191–5.

37. Faure S, de Santa Barbara P. Molecular embryology of the foregut. J Pediatr Gastroenterol Nutr 2011; 52(Suppl 1):S2–3.

38. Murakami G, Sato I, Shimada K, et al. Direct lymphatic drainage from the esophagus into the thoracic duct. Surg Radiol Anat 1994;16:399–407.

39. Rice TW, Bronner MP. The esophageal wall. Thorac Surg Clin 2011;21:299–305.

40. Saito H, Sato T, Miyazaki M. Extramural lymphatic drainage from the thoracic esophagus based on minute cadaveric dissections: fundamentals for the sentinel node navigation surgery for the thoracic esophageal cancers. Surg Radiol Anat 2007;29:532–42.

41. Riquet M, Le Pimbec Barthes F, Souilamas R, et al. Thoracic duct tributaries from intrathoracic organs. Ann Thorac Surg 2002;73:892–8 [discussion: 898–9].

42. Kuge K, Murakani G, Mizobuchi S, et al. Submucosal territory of the direct lymphatic drainage system to the thoracic duct in the human esophagus. J Thorac Cardiovasc Surg 2003;125:1343–9.

43. Riquet M, Hidden G, Debesse B. Abdominal nodal connexions of the lymphatics of the lungs. Surg Radiol Anat 1988;10:251–2.

44. Meyer KK. Direct lymphatic connections from the lower lobes of the lung to the abdomen. J Thorac Surg 1958;356:726–33.

45. Caplan I. Anatomical review of the lymph nodes of the human mediastinum. Surg Radiol Anat 1990;12:9–18.

46. Le Pimbec Barthes F, Riquet M, Hartl D, et al. Cervical venous anastomosis of pulmonary lymphatic vessels. Surg Radiol Anat 1997;19:53–5.

47. Naruke T, Suemasu K, Ishikawa S. Lymph node mapping and curability of various levels of metastases in resected lung cancer. J Thorac Cardiovasc Surg 1978;76:832–9.

48. Mountain CF, Dresler CM. Regional lymph node classification for lung cancer staging. Chest 1997; 111:1718–23.

49. Skandalakis JE, Skandalakis LI, Skandalakis PN. Anatomy of the lymphatics. Surg Oncol Clin N Am 2007;16:1–16.

50. Jdanov DA. Anatomy of the thoracic duct and of the main lymphatic vessels of the trunk in man. Acta Anat (Basel) 1959;37:20–47.

51. Kinnaert P. Anatomical variations of the cervical part of the thoracic duct in man. J Anat 1973;115:45–52.

52. Langford RJ, Daudia AT, Malins TJ. A morphological study of the thoracic duct at the jugulo-subclavian junction. J Craniomaxillofac Surg 1999;27:100–4.

53. Murakami G, Abe M, Abe T. Last-intercalated node and direct lymphatic drainage into the thoracic duct from the thoraco-abdominal viscera. Jpn J Thorac Cardiovasc Surg 2002;50:93–103.

Computed Tomography and Magnetic Resonance Imaging of the Thoracic Lymphatic System

Maria Luisa Mennini, MD, Carlo Catalano, MD*,
Maurizio Del Monte, MD, Francesco Fraioli, MD

KEYWORDS

- Computed tomography • Magnetic resonance imaging
- Lung cancer • Lymph nodes

Various noninvasive diagnostic techniques, such as chest radiography, computed tomography (CT), positron emission tomography (PET), and magnetic resonance imaging (MRI), are currently available for assessing intrathoracic nodal status.[1]

The lymph nodes distributed through the mediastinum and hila are best understood by correlation with CT and magnetic resonance (MR) cross-sectional images.[2,3] In particular, imaging of mediastinal or hilar lymph node disorders includes enlargement and abnormal density on chest radiographs, attenuation on CT, or signal intensity on MRI. However, it is necessary to consider very carefully the risk that sometimes lymph nodes of normal attenuation or signal intensity can harbor malignancy.[4,5]

The characterization of enlarged mediastinal lymph nodes is crucial for staging and prognosis as well as for treatment planning.

Eighty percent of lung cancers are non–small cell lung cancers (NSCLC); for this histologic subtype, prognosis and management are strongly related to the involvement of hilar and mediastinal lymph nodes.[4,6] Surgical resection or induction therapy is planned almost exclusively on the basis of the lymph node status. The presence of nodal metastases limits therapeutic options and also indicates a worse prognosis.[4,6] Thus, it becomes crucial to obtain this information before therapy.

However, mediastinal lymph node involvement can also be a manifestation of Hodgkin disease, non-Hodgkin lymphoma, infection, metastases from organs other than the lung, sarcoidosis, and other disorders, both localized and systemic (**Box 1**).

CHEST RADIOGRAPHY

In current clinical practice, the first imaging study done in a patient with suspected lung cancer with or without mediastinal or hilar metastatic lesions is usually chest radiography.

It is often difficult to assess the mediastinum using standard chest radiography. The site and number of involved lymph node stations are visualized; also, information about density (solid, fatty, fluid) should be obtained if possible. This radiographic examination is certainly more accurate in evaluating the primary lesion and the potential association with pleural involvement. Digitalized imaging strongly contributes to improving the accuracy of this examination. Old radiographs, if available, are often helpful for comparison.

The radiologic findings suggesting hilar lymph node enlargement include enlargement of the

Department of Radiological Sciences, "Sapienza" University of Rome, Policlinico Umberto I, V.le Regina Elena 324, Roma 00161, Italy
* Corresponding author.
E-mail address: carlo.catalano@uniroma1.it

Thorac Surg Clin 22 (2012) 155–160
doi:10.1016/j.thorsurg.2011.12.009

Box 1
Causes of mediastinal and hilar lymph node enlargement

Infectious
- Common
  Primary tuberculosis
  Fungal infection
- Uncommon
  Viral
  Bacterial

Inflammatory
- Sarcoidosis
- Silicosis
- Coal worker's pneumoconiosis
- Asbestosis
- Wegener granulomatosis
- Interstitial pneumonia
- Collagen vascular disease

Neoplasm
- Primary
  Lymphoma
  Leukemia
  Myeloma
- Metastatic

Other
- Reactive hyperplasia
- Castleman disease
- Amyloidosis
- Whipple disease
- Chronic eosinophilic pneumonia
- Chronic congestive heart failure
- Drug-induced lymphadenopathy

---

these techniques show superior contrast resolution, they are also performed to characterize the tissue components of the mass. These techniques are in particular useful to distinguish vascular lesions resulting from benign disorders of the mediastinum, such as lipomatosis, from potential malignant pathologic conditions warranting further investigation.[7–9]

CT is usually performed to assess and characterize mediastinal masses located in the anterior and middle mediastinum. MRI is usually performed to evaluate masses located in the posterior compartment: most of these masses turn out to be neurogenic, arising from the sympathetic ganglia or from the nerve roots. In such cases, MRI can also clearly depict spinal involvement.[10] MRI is also extremely useful to evaluate the thoracic inlet.

CT

Historically, CT has been used as the primary diagnostic imaging modality to assess and stage mediastinal and hilar lymph nodes; this technique has been performed merely on the basis of size criteria. However, tissue density and extracapsular involvement are also considered. Sensitivity, specificity, and accuracy are strongly improved by the use of a variety of nonaxial plane reconstructions, including coronal and sagittal views, as well as several angled planes and volume rendering.[9,10] Scans are usually obtained from the lung apex to the diaphragm during suspended inspiration. Scanning parameters at multidetector -row CT could be: 120–140 kV, 330 mA, 1 mm collimation and 3 mm slice thickness, with no interslice gap. CT scans after injection of contrast medium are obtained with a scan delay of 30 to 40 seconds. The multidetector spiral technique has further improved the ability of CT to study the mediastinum by markedly shortening the scanning time, limiting respiratory motion artifacts, and reducing the dose of iodinated contrast.

Lymphadenopathy

In CT images, enlarged hilar or mediastinal nodes are usually seen as round or oval soft tissue lesions (**Fig. 1**). The use of size alone in CT scan as a parameter to predict malignancy in lung cancer is fraught with error. Multicriteria evaluation is mandatory. A short-axis diameter lesser than 10 mm, nodular calcifications, and intranodal fat tissue are criteria for the mass to be considered benign. Focal low density other than fat suggesting necrosis, invasion of surrounding mediastinal fat, hilar lymph nodes with convex margins bulging toward the surrounding pulmonary parenchyma, and coalescence of adjacent and enlarged nodes

---

hilum, increased lobulation of hilar contours, presence of a rounded mass in a portion of the hilum that does not contain major vessels, and increased density of the hilum itself.

However, once a mediastinal or hilar abnormality is detected or suspected on plain chest radiography, cross-sectional CT imaging is mandatory.

CT AND MRI OF THE THORACIC LYMPHATIC SYSTEM

CT or MRI is used to assess the location and extent of primary and secondary lesions. Because

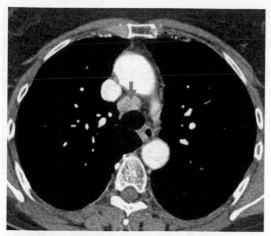

Fig. 1. Mediastinal lymphadenopathy. Contrast-enhanced CT with mediastinal window settings reveals lymphadenopathy in the precarinal region (*arrow*). After transbronchial needle aspiration, the diagnosis was metastatic adenocarcinoma.

forming larger masses are considered as criteria for malignancy.[11–13]

The recognition of hilar node enlargement by CT is facilitated by intravenous contrast opacification of the hilar vessels; in fact, CT after intravenous administration of contrast material can help in distinguishing vessels from lymph nodes in doubtful cases, depicting vascular abnormalities or small masses that do not deform the mediastinal contours on chest radiographs.

CT may also be used as a semi-invasive technique for direct guidance of biopsy of enlarged mediastinal lymph nodes and, in experimental studies, for indirect virtual guidance of transbronchial needle aspiration.[14,15]

Lymph node calcifications and high attenuation seen on CT

CT demonstrates the presence of lymph node calcifications much better than standard chest radiography. High attenuation usually means that the density is higher than that of a muscle (>60 Hounsfield units [HU]).

Lymph node calcifications can be seen in benign conditions such as sarcoidosis (punctate pattern, bilateral and diffuse involvement in the III–IV stage), Castleman disease, or infectious diseases such as tuberculosis (the node is completely calcified and usually unilateral).

Lymph node calcifications are rarely due to neoplastic disease; however, osteosarcoma, chondrosarcoma, carcinoids, and mucinous carcinoma may rarely show these patterns; past medical history helps to direct diagnosis.

Lymph node calcifications can also occur after treatment of mediastinal lymphoma, both with chemotherapy and radiotherapy.

Thin peripheral calcifications (eggshell calcifications) of a part of the node can be seen in patients with coal worker's pneumoconiosis, silicosis, and sarcoidosis.[16–19]

Low attenuation on CT (about −20 to +20 HU)

Enlarged nodes with internal areas of low CT attenuation (density higher than fat but lower than that of muscle) would likely contain areas of internal necrosis; this condition can be seen in a variety of diseases, including tuberculosis, atypical manifestations of atypical mycobacteriosis, abscess, Whipple disease, and neoplastic disorders.

Many tumors can undergo cystic degeneration, especially after radiation therapy or chemotherapy.

In a CT scan, a prominent fatty hilum sign is associated with benign diseases, typically resulting from previous inflammation. However, obliteration of the fatty hilum may be associated with metastatic disease, particularly testicular tumors and lymphoma.[20–22]

Contrast-enhanced CT

Moderate increase in attenuation after contrast administration is observed in enlarged mediastinal nodes of patients affected by tuberculosis, fungal infections, sarcoidosis, and metastatic lesions. When contrast enhancement is significant, it suggests metastatic disease from a highly vascular primary tumor, such as melanoma, parathyroid or thyroid carcinoma, carcinoid tumor, renal cancer, hemangioma, or leiomyosarcoma. Castleman disease is a rare cause of markedly contrast-enhanced lymph nodes.[23–26]

MRI

MRI of the chest is a powerful evolving tool for scientific and clinical application.[27]

The recent development of MR parallel imaging techniques allowed the acquisition of diffusion-weighted MRI (DWI) of the body; DWI has also been recently applied to characterize lung carcinomas and mediastinal lymph nodes.[28]

MRI of the lung has been considered experimental for many years; combining fast breath-hold acquisitions with parallel imaging, rotating phase encoding, and navigator technology, lung MRI has become a fairly robust technique with broad clinical applications.[29] The development of fast imaging techniques in combination with parallel imaging has also allowed the integration of DWI in morphologic chest MRI without image degradation due to motion artifacts.[30]

Table 1
Sequences for lung MRI

Sequence	Key Pathology	Respiration Maneuver	Spatial Resolution	Temporal Resolution	1.5 T	3 T
STIR T2 or propeller	Lymph node/bone metastases	Multiple breath holds	Moderate	Low	+	+
T2 propeller	Nodules and masses	Multiple breath holds	Moderate	Moderate	+	+
T2 propeller T2 TSE rt*	Masses	Free breathing	Moderate–high	Low	+	+
DWI	Nodules and masses	Multiple breath holds	Low	Low	+	+

Abbreviations: rt, respiratory triggered; STIR, short tau inversion recovery.

Diffusion-weighted MR images can map the signal that reflects the microscopic movement of water molecules (Brownian motion) in the examined tissue.[31] Brownian motion can also be measured as signal loss and expressed as an apparent diffusion coefficient value with the use of diffusion-sensitive sequences. DWI detects abnormalities on the basis of tumor cellularity. Tumors are more cellular than the tissue from which they originate; thus, they would show a relatively high signal intensity on DWI.[32]

Preliminary results have shown that DWI has a high negative predictive value to exclude mediastinal lymph node metastases from NSCLC and can potentially be a reliable noninvasive imaging alternative in the preoperative staging of mediastinal lymph nodes in patients with NSCLC.[33]

MRI is the primary imaging modality to evaluate mediastinal abnormalities that are suspected to be vascular. MRI and CT provide comparable information for size assessment of enlarged mediastinal nodes.[34] For these reasons, MRI is currently performed primarily in patients with a contraindication to the intravenous administration of iodinated contrast material.

New pulse sequences such as DWI sequence are currently under investigation, and recently they have also been shown to be more accurate than fludeoxyglucose F 18 PET for mediastinal nodal staging in patients with lung cancer.[35]

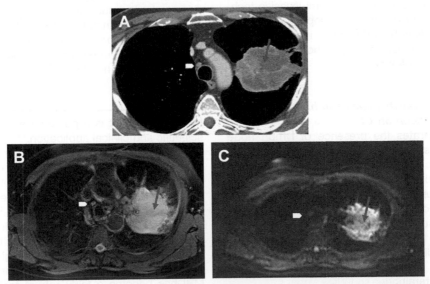

Fig. 2. A 65-year-old woman with NSCLC. (*A*) Contrast-enhanced CT with mediastinal window settings reveals a left neoplastic mass (*arrow*) with lymphadenopathy in the right paratracheal region (*arrowhead*). (*B*) Transverse electrocardiographically triggered and respiratory-triggered T2-weighted image confirms a 7-cm mass in the left upper lobe (*arrow*) and a 1-cm right paratracheal lymph node (*arrowhead*) that does not meet the size criteria for metastasis. (*C*) DWI sequence with b value of 250 shows an area of high signal intensity in the paratracheal region suggesting micrometastatic disease (*arrowhead*); the left lung tumor mass was confirmed (*arrow*).

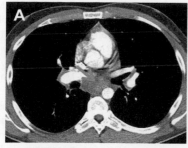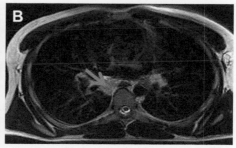

Fig. 3. (*A*) Contrast-enhanced CT shows the presence of enlarged subcarinal lymph nodes (*arrow*). (*B*) Transverse electrocardiographically triggered and respiratory-triggered T2-weighted image confirms the subcarinal mass (*arrow*). Biopsy allowed the diagnosis of lymphoma.

MRI can provide better tissue characterization than CT; it confirms the cystic nature of mediastinal lesions that may appear solid on CT, such as bronchogenic cysts; it may also demonstrate vascular structures in patients who are unable to undergo contrast CT. Two potential disadvantages of MRI, when compared with CT, are poor depiction of calcification and comparatively poorer spatial resolution.[36]

Hilar node enlargement may be more easily recognized by MRI than noncontrast CT.

All MRI examinations can be performed with a 1.5/3-T clinical imager by using a body-phased array coil (**Table 1**).

Before DWI and short tau inversion recovery MRI, T1- and T2-weighted images are obtained in the transverse plane; transverse diffusion-weighted MR images are obtained with b values of 50 and 1000 s/mm². Quantitative analysis of diffusion-weighted MR images allows better assessment of metastatic lymphadenopathies. In DWI, mediastinal metastatic spreading is defined as a focus of low signal intensity at the site of a visible lymph node on the corresponding T2-weighted image regardless of its size.

For T1-weighted images, a 3-dimensional multishot gradient-recalled echo sequence with breath holds may be used to measure nodal size on short-axis morphologic details (eccentric cortical thickening or obliterated fatty hilum) of mediastinal nodal metastasis shown on T2-weighted (fast-spin echo [FSE]) images.[37]

On T2-weighted triple-inversion black-blood FSE MRI, malignant nodes show high signal intensity with obliterated fatty hilum or eccentric cortical thickening.

Benign lymph nodes show low signal intensity or typical fatty hilum.[38]

MRI may help to differentiate between benign and malignant lymph nodes by showing low signal intensity on T2-weighted imaging and hilar node enlargement; these parameters can be more easily evaluated by MRI than noncontrast CT (**Figs. 2 and 3**).

MRI of the chest allows detection and characterization of a large range of mediastinal disorders. With fast-growing experience in the application of MRI, this technique could play an important role in future diagnostic set-up of many mediastinal diseases, especially in younger patients.[39]

REFERENCES

1. Ettinger DS. Overview and state of the art in the management of lung cancer. Oncology (Williston Park) 2004;18(7 Suppl 4):7–9.
2. Dooms GC, Hricak H, Crooks LE, et al. Magnetic resonance imaging of the lymph nodes: comparison with CT. Radiology 1984;153:719–28.
3. McLoud TC, Bourgouin PM, Greenberg RW, et al. Bronchogenic carcinoma: analysis of staging in the mediastinum with CT by correlative lymph node mapping and sampling. Radiology 1992;182:319–23.
4. Schaefer-Prokop C, Prokop M. New imaging techniques in the treatment guidelines for lung cancer. Eur Respir J 2002;35:71s–83s.
5. Webb WR, Sarin M, Zerhouni EA, et al. Interobserver variability in CT and MR staging of lung cancer. J Comput Assist Tomogr 1993;17:841–6.
6. Shim SS, Lee KS, Kim BT, et al. Non-small cell lung cancer: prospective comparison of integrated FDG PET/CT and CT alone for preoperative staging. Radiology 2005;236:1009–11.
7. Musset D, Grenier P, Carette MF, et al. Primary lung cancer staging: prospective comparative study of MR imaging with CT. Radiology 1986;160:607–11.
8. Glazer GM, Orringer MB, Gross BH, et al. The mediastinum in non-small cell lung cancer: CT-surgical correlation. AJR Am J Roentgenol 1984;142:1101–5.
9. Martini N, Heelan R, Westcott J, et al. Comparative merits of conventional, computed tomographic, and magnetic resonance imaging in assessing mediastinal involvement in surgically confirmed lung carcinoma. J Thorac Cardiovasc Surg 1985;90:639–48.

10. Poon PY, Bronskill MJ, Henkelman RM, et al. Mediastinal lymph node metastases from bronchogenic carcinoma: detection with MR imaging and CT. Radiology 1987;162:651–6.

11. Passlick B, Izbicki JR, Kubuschok B, et al. Detection of disseminated lung cancer cells in lymph nodes: impact on staging and prognosis. Ann Thorac Surg 1996;61:177–82.

12. Chabbert V, Canevet G, Baixas C, et al. Mediastinal lymphadenopathy in congestive heart failure: a sequential CT evaluation with clinical and echocardiographic correlations. Eur Radiol 2004;14:881–9.

13. Seely JM, Mayo JR, Miller RR, et al. T1 lung cancer: prevalence of mediastinal lymph node metastases and diagnostic accuracy of CT. Radiology 1993; 186:129–32.

14. Laurent F, Drouillard J, Dorcier F, et al. Bronchogenic carcinoma staging: CT versus MR imaging. Assessment with surgery. Eur J Cardiothorac Surg 1988;2:31–6.

15. Wahl RL, Quint LE, Greenough RL, et al. Staging of mediastinal non-small cell lung cancer with FDG-PET, CT, and fusion images: preliminary prospective evaluation. Radiology 1994;191:371–7.

16. Sussman SK, Halvorsen RA Jr, Silverman PM, et al. Paracardiac adenopathy: CT evaluation. Am J Roentgenol 1987;149:29–34.

17. Niimi H, Kang EY, Kwong JS, et al. CT of chronic infiltrative lung disease: prevalence of mediastinal lymphadenopathy. J Comput Assist Tomogr 1996;20:305–8.

18. Thomas RD, Blaquiere RM. Reactive mediastinal lymphadenopathy in bronchiectasis assessed by CT. Acta Radiol 1993;34:489–91.

19. Boiselle PM, Patz EF Jr, Vining DJ, et al. Imaging of mediastinal lymph nodes: CT, MR, and FDG PET. Radiographics 1998;18:1061–9.

20. Slanetz PJ, Truong M, Shepard JA, et al. Mediastinal lymphadenopathy and hazy mediastinal fat: new CT findings of congestive heart failure. AJR Am J Roentgenol 1998;171:1307–9.

21. Ngom A, Dumont P, Diot P, et al. Benign mediastinal lymphadenopathy in congestive heart failure. Chest 2001;119:653–6.

22. Erly WK, Borders RJ, Outwater EK, et al. Location, size, and distribution of mediastinal lymph node enlargement in chronic congestive heart failure. J Comput Assist Tomogr 2003;27:485–9.

23. Armstrong P. Mediastinal and hilar disorders. In: Armstrong P, Wilson AG, Dee P, et al, editors. Imaging of diseases of the chest. London: Mosby; 2000. p. 789–892.

24. McAdams HP, Kirejczyk WM, Rosado-de-Christenson ML, et al. Bronchogenic cyst: imaging features with clinical and histopathologic correlation. Radiology 2000;217:441–6.

25. Kawashima A, Fishman EK, Kuhlman JE, et al. CT of the posterior mediastinal masses. Radiographics 1991;11:1045–67.

26. McAdams HP, Rosado-de-Christenson ML, Moran CA. Mediastinal hemangioma: radiographic and CT features in 4 patients. Radiology 1994;193:399–402.

27. Boiselle PM. MR imaging of thoracic lymph nodes. A comparison of computed tomography and positron emission tomography. Magn Reson Imaging Clin N Am 2000;8:33–41.

28. Mori T, Nomori H, Ikeda K, et al. Diffusion-weighted magnetic resonance imaging for diagnosing malignant pulmonary nodules/masses: comparison with positron emission tomography. J Thorac Oncol 2008;3:358–64.

29. Ohno Y, Sugimura K, Hatabu H. MR imaging of lung cancer. Eur J Radiol 2002;44:172–81.

30. Ohno Y, Koyama H, Onishi Y, et al. Non-small cell lung cancer: whole body MR examination for M-stage assessment—utility for whole-body diffusion-weighted imaging compared with integrated FDG PET/CT. Radiology 2008;248:643–54.

31. Matoba M, Tonami H, Kondou T, et al. Lung carcinoma: diffusion-weighted MR imaging—preliminary evaluation with apparent diffusion coefficient. Radiology 2007;243:570–7.

32. Takenaka D, Ohno Y, Hatabu H, et al. Differentiation of metastatic versus non-metastatic mediastinal lymph nodes in patients with non-small cell lung cancer using respiratory-triggered short inversion time inversion recovery (STIR) turbo spin-echo MR imaging. Eur J Radiol 2002;44:216–24.

33. Koh DM, Collins DJ. Diffusion-weighted MRI in the body: applications and challenges in oncology. Am J Roentgenol 2007;188:1622–35.

34. Abdel Razek AA, Soliman NY, Elkhamary S, et al. Role of diffusion weighted MR imaging in cervical lymphadenopathy. Eur Radiol 2006;16:1468–77.

35. Fujimoto K, Edamitsu O, Meno S, et al. [MR diagnosis for metastasis or non-metastasis of mediastinal and hilar lymph nodes in cases of primary lung cancer: detectability, signal intensity, and MR-pathologic correlation]. Nippon Acta Radiol 1995; 55:162–71 [in Japanese].

36. Walker R, Kessar P, Blanchard R, et al. Turbo STIR magnetic resonance imaging as a whole-body screening tool for metastases in patients with breast carcinoma: preliminary clinical experience. J Magn Reson Imaging 2000;11:343–50.

37. Eustase S, Tello R, DeCarvalho V, et al. Whole body turbo STIR MRI in unknown primary tumor detection. J Magn Reson Imaging 1998;8:751–3.

38. Ohno Y, Hatabu H, Takenaka D, et al. Metastases in mediastinal and hilar lymph nodes in patients with non-small cell lung cancer: quantitative and qualitative assessment with STIR turbo spin-echo MR imaging. Radiology 2004;231:872–9.

39. Leung DA, Debatin JF. Three-dimensional contrast enhanced magnetic resonance angiography of the thoracic vasculature. Eur Radiol 1997;7:981–9.

PET Staging of Mediastinal Lymph Nodes in Thoracic Oncology

Stephen R. Broderick, MD, Bryan F. Meyers, MD, MPH*

KEYWORDS

- Non–small cell lung cancer • Esophageal cancer • FDG-PET
- PET-CT • Staging

Positron emission tomography (PET), an imaging modality based on the metabolic activity of tissues, has been developed during the last two decades. As applied in oncology, this technology takes advantage of the relatively high rate of cellular glucose uptake and glycolysis in malignant cells compared with normal cells. In PET imaging, the radiolabeled glucose analog ^{18}F-flouro-2-deoxy-D-glucose (FDG) is administered intravenously to patients. FDG undergoes the same cellular uptake as glucose and is phosphorylated by hexokinase generating ^{18}F-FDG-6-phosphate. Because of the increased uptake of FDG and decreased rate of dephosphorylation in malignant cells, this radiolabeled metabolite accumulates in malignant cells and can be imaged with a PET camera.

Standardized quantitative criteria for abnormal PET findings are lacking. Comparison of FDG uptake in a target area with surrounding tissue or normal lung or liver provides a qualitative assessment of PET activity. A semiquantitative parameter, the standardized uptake value (SUV), is roughly the ratio of FDG in the tissue of interest compared with normal uptake. A value of less than 2.5 is often considered normal, but this parameter is subject to variation across scanners, centers, and interpreting physicians. The attempted use of PET to differentiate malignant and benign lesions has become commonplace. However, results can be either false-positive in patients with infectious or inflammatory lesions or false-negative in patients with slow-growing or low-grade malignancies.

There is an extensive and growing body of literature about the role of PET in the management of non–small cell lung cancer (NSCLC) and esophageal cancer. This article focuses on the use of PET in mediastinal staging of these common thoracic malignancies. A review of the evidence for and against the use of PET in mediastinal staging is provided and the use of PET in practice is discussed.

NON–SMALL CELL LUNG CANCER

PET scanning has become an essential part of the initial evaluation of patients with suspected NSCLC. It is useful in discriminating between benign and malignant solitary pulmonary nodules, and in the identification of extrathoracic spread of disease. There exists an extensive body of literature on these uses of PET in NSCLC, discussion of which is beyond the scope of this article.

Accurate staging of mediastinal lymph nodes is essential to management of NSCLC. Evaluation of mediastinal lymph nodes for metastatic disease allows for selection of patients for stage-based therapy and provides patients with the best estimate of prognosis. In the absence of distant metastatic disease, the status of mediastinal lymph nodes is a primary determinant of resectability and the main driver of additional preresection staging. Patients without evidence of disease in

Division of Cardiothoracic Surgery, Department of Surgery, Washington University School of Medicine, 3108 Queeny Tower, One Barnes-Jewish Hospital Plaza, St. Louis, MO 63110-1013, USA
* Corresponding author.
E-mail address: meyersb@wustl.edu

Thorac Surg Clin 22 (2012) 161–166
doi:10.1016/j.thorsurg.2011.12.004
1547-4127/12/$ – see front matter © 2012 Elsevier Inc. All rights reserved.

mediastinal N2 nodes are generally considered candidates for primary resection, whereas those with N2 lymph node metastases are treated with neoadjuvant therapy and surgery, or definitive chemotherapy or radiotherapy.

PET has become an important modality and is now routinely used for mediastinal lymph node staging in NSCLC. Before the advent of PET, noninvasive staging of mediastinal nodes was performed using computed tomography (CT) to look at the diameter of lymph nodes as a predictor of their malignant or benign nature. The accuracy of CT alone in identifying metastatic disease to mediastinal lymph nodes is poor, with approximate sensitivity and specificity of 50% and 85%, respectively.[1] The use of PET, and subsequently combined PET-CT, in staging the mediastinum has been evaluated in many studies during the past 15 years, including several prospective, randomized, controlled trials.

An important randomized trial to evaluate the effectiveness of PET in mediastinal staging of NSCLC was the PLUS trial.[2] The PLUS trial randomized 188 patients with suspected NSCLC who were scheduled for surgery to one of two arms: conventional staging work-up or conventional staging work-up with the addition of PET. The primary end point was the number of "futile" thoracotomies, a term crafted for the study and defined as thoracotomy for benign disease, an exploratory thoracotomy without resection, the detection of pathologic N2 disease at resection, or either recurrence or death within 12 months of surgery. In the conventional staging work-up arm, 41% (39 of 96) of patients had futile thoracotomy compared with only 21% (19 of 92) with the addition of PET to the staging evaluation. The authors concluded that the addition of PET to conventional staging work-up resulted in a 51% relative reduction in the number of futile thoracotomies and prevented unnecessary surgery in one of five patients with suspected NSCLC.

In 2003 The American College of Surgeons Oncology Group published the results of the Z0050 trial.[3] This prospective trial enrolled 303 patients from 22 institutions with documented or suspected NSCLC deemed resectable after completion of standard staging procedures. The primary end point of this study was to determine whether the addition of PET after standard work-up identified lesions that precluded curative pulmonary resection. In comparison with the PLUS trial, the Z0050 trial included a substantially smaller proportion of patients with locally advanced (IIIA–IIIB) disease and radiographic staging including CT of the chest and upper abdomen, bone scintigraphy, and CT or MRI of

the head was required before PET. The results of the Z0050 trial paralleled those of the PLUS trial. PET applied after a negative conventional work-up identified unresectable disease in 43 (14.2%) of 303 patients and nontherapeutic thoracotomy was avoided in one of five patients.

Viney and colleagues[4] published a randomized controlled trial investigating the role of PET in NSCLC in 2004. This study was limited to patients with suspected clinical stage I to II disease. In contrast to PLUS and Z0050, this study did not demonstrate a reduction in the number of thoracotomies performed in patients undergoing PET scan preoperatively. However, PET suggested a change in stage in 18% of patients, predominantly by identifying previously unsuspected occult N2 disease. The approach to patients with stage IIIa disease at the centers performing this study at the time was primary surgery. Therefore, the identification of N2 disease by PET would not have affected the end point of number of thoracotomies performed. The authors of the study acknowledge that had their treatment algorithm for stage IIIa (N2) NSCLC involved neoadjuvant or definitive chemotherapy rather than primary surgery, PET imaging may have altered therapy by preventing thoracotomy in up to 20% of patients. It is clear from these high-quality studies that the information from PET adds a substantial amount of staging knowledge in patients with resectable lung cancer.

PET imaging provides information regarding the metabolic activity of a lesion. The precise location of focal PET abnormalities is difficult to interpret. In contrast, CT imaging provides detailed anatomic imaging without information on the metabolic activity of a lesion. Integrated PET-CT became clinically available in 2000,[5] with the presumed advantage of more accurately correlating metabolic activity with precise anatomic locations. It is quite probable that the enhanced value of PET-CT might have leveraged the staging advantages of PET even further, had it been available for those early trials described in the preceding paragraphs.

The diagnostic accuracy of integrated PET-CT has been compared with that of CT alone, PET alone, and visual correlation of CT and PET by Lardinois and colleagues[6] in 2003. In this prospective study of 50 patients with known or suspected NSCLC integrated PET-CT correctly staged the mediastinum of 5 of 11 patients who were incorrectly staged by conventional correlation of PET and CT, indicating that integrated PET-CT improved the accuracy of staging in NSCLC. This finding was confirmed by Cerfolio and colleagues[7] in 2004 who demonstrated that PET-CT had a higher sensitivity, specificity, and positive predictive value for N2 disease compared with PET alone. The use of PET-CT in staging was subsequently evaluated in two randomized clinical trials.

In 2009, Fischer and colleagues[8] randomized 189 patients to conventional staging or conventional staging plus integrated PET-CT. In that study, 94% of patients underwent mediastinoscopy. The primary end point of the study was the number of futile thoracotomies performed, defined as a thoracotomy performed for stage IIIA or higher disease or a benign lesion, exploratory thoracotomy, or thoracotomy in a patient who suffered recurrence of disease or death from any cause within 12 months of surgery. Sixty thoracotomies were performed in the PET-CT group, 21 of which were characterized as futile. In comparison, 73 thoracotomies were performed in the conventional staging group, 38 of which were labeled as futile. In total, 21 (21%) of 98 patients in the PET-CT group underwent futile thoracotomy compared with 38 (42%) of 91 patients in the conventional staging group, results that remarkably mirror the outcome of the PLUS study, described previously. As the PLUS and American College of Surgeons Oncology Group Z0050 trials demonstrated for stand-alone PET, this study demonstrated that integrated PET-CT improved sensitivity of preoperative mediastinal staging in NSCLC. For every five PET-CT scans performed, one futile thoracotomy was avoided. Reassurance about the effects of the randomization in this trial is seen by the fact that the number of justified thoracotomies and survival were similar between the groups. Also in 2009, Maziak and colleagues[9] published the results of the Early Lung PET trial (ELPET), a clinical trial comparing PET-CT plus cranial imaging with conventional (non-PET) staging with cranial imaging. This study randomized 337 patients and similarly found that PET-CT correctly upstaged a significant proportion of patients by identifying N2 or extrathoracic disease. However, in approximately 5% of patients who underwent PET-CT, disease was incorrectly upstaged with false-positive findings.

Although PET-CT may prevent nontherapeutic thoracotomies by identifying unrecognized N2 disease, false-positive N2 disease, if accepted without confirmation, has the potential to deprive possibly resectable patients of curative surgery. A recently published subgroup analysis of the ELPET trial confirms the need for pathologic confirmation of mediastinal abnormalities identified on PET-CT.[10] In the ELPET trial, 149 patients underwent PET-CT and subsequent mediastinoscopy or thoracotomy with lymph node sampling.

The sensitivity and specificity of PET-CT for N2 disease was 70% and 94%, respectively. Mediastinal N2 disease was identified by PET-CT in 22 patients, eight of whom did not have pathologically identifiable tumor in the mediastinum. If invasive mediastinal staging had not been pursued, these eight patients would have either been deprived of potentially curative surgery or inappropriately subjected to induction therapy, emphasizing the need for pathologic confirmation of abnormalities identified on PET-CT.

In light of its ability to prevent unnecessary surgery by the identification of previously unidentified N2 disease, it is common practice in North America to obtain routine PET-CT or PET scanning in patients with clinical stage I to IIIA NSCLC before resection. Pathologic confirmation of N2 disease identified on PET by endobronchial ultrasound (EBUS), endoscopic ultrasound (EUS), or mediastinoscopy is advised to avoid inappropriate treatment decisions based on false-positive results. Although the evidence is not fully presented in this article, one might also recommend that invasive mediastinal staging be pursued in patients in whom clinical suspicion of N2 disease is high, despite negative evaluation on PET or PET-CT. It is certainly possible that the value of PET or PET-CT in mediastinal staging is variable depending on the country or region in which it is taking place. The prevalence and severity of infectious or granulomatous diseases, such as histoplasmosis or tuberculosis, will alter the "background noise" in a population and thus alter the definition of a positive or negative study. Work is in progress by Grogan and colleagues at Vanderbilt University to examine the impact of this phenomenon of local and regional differences in the value of PET.

ESOPHAGEAL CANCER

As in lung cancer, accurate staging of esophageal cancer is essential to offer stage-appropriate therapy and provide information regarding prognosis to patients and their physicians. The role of PET and PET-CT in staging mediastinal lymph nodes in esophageal cancer is less well-defined than in NSCLC.

An early investigation into the role of PET in staging of esophageal cancer was performed at Washington University in St. Louis and published in 1997. In the initial study PET and CT imaging was performed in 29 patients with biopsy-proved esophageal cancer.[11] Seven of 29 patients were suspected to have metastatic disease at the time of surgery and underwent only confirmatory tissue sampling rather than resection. PET identified five of these seven patients, whereas CT scan was negative in all of them. In a subsequent update to that experience, in patients who were deemed clinically operable 17 of 52 had distant metastatic disease identified by PET, precluding resection.[12] CT detected metastatic disease in only 5 of the 17 patients. In addition, pathologic examination identified lymph node metastases in 21 patients, 11 of which were identified by PET compared with 6 by CT. In a similar study from the University of Pittsburgh, PET demonstrated increased uptake outside of the primary tumor in 18 of 35 patients considered to have resectable disease.[13] Sixteen of 18 patients had true-positive findings including locoregional and distant metastases. In subsequent years, multiple small studies evaluated the role of PET in the clinical evaluation of esophageal cancer and demonstrated that PET was more sensitive than CT in identifying distant metastatic spread of disease.[14] The use of PET in identifying locoregional spread of disease is less clear. The common wisdom is that the bright signal from the primary tumor potentially obscures less intense FDG uptake in nearby lymph nodes, thus rendering PET less useful for the identification of nodal metastases.

In 1999, the American College of Surgeons Oncology Group began accrual to the Z0060 trial.[15] This was a prospective multi-institutional study designed to evaluate whether the addition of PET detected metastatic disease that would preclude surgery in patients deemed operable after conventional staging. The objective of the study was to determine whether PET could identify more than 5% of patients with unresectable disease before resection, thereby avoiding unnecessary surgery. A total of 262 patients with biopsy-proved carcinoma were enrolled after CT scan of the chest and abdomen demonstrated no evidence of metastatic disease. A total of 199 patients were eligible for the study and 189 of these were evaluable. PET scan was suggestive of M1b disease that was subsequently confirmed in nine patients (4.8%). In an additional 9.5% of patients, M1b disease was suggested by PET but histologic confirmation was not pursued, suggesting that PET identified previously unrecognized disease in greater than 5% of patients. Notably, two patients were identified to have extensive N1 disease on preoperative PET scan precluding operation.

There were several factors confounding interpretation of the Z0060 trial. One factor was the inclusion of patients with very early cancer into the trial. Even patients with microscopic adenocarcinoma arising from flat Barrett esophagus were allowed inclusion, and this cohort of patients is highly unlikely to benefit from a more extensive metastatic evaluation. Technical advances in PET scanning and the introduction of integrated PET-CT during the accrual phase may mean that the use of PET demonstrated in the Z0060 study is an underestimate of what is currently possible. Three recent studies have demonstrated superior assessment of nodal metastases in esophageal cancer by integrated PET-CT compared with CT alone or CT combined with stand-alone PET.[16–18] A protocol amendment during accrual allowed for the administration of induction therapy to study subjects provided their PET scan was obtained before therapy. With regard to locoregional disease, patients with extensive N1 disease on PET could lead to selection of a strategy of induction or definitive chemotherapy rather than surgical resection. Because some patients undergoing induction therapy may not ultimately come to resection, the evaluation of the ability of PET to identify nodal metastases may be underestimated in Z0060. The use of EUS was sporadic during early enrollment in the trial but had become commonplace by 2004 when enrollment concluded. Findings on EUS suggestive of advanced T stage or N1 or M1a disease would often lead to induction therapy despite negative findings on PET evaluation. Although Z0060 showed that PET-identified nodal disease altered treatment strategy in a small number of patients, the development of EUS and EUS-guided fine-needle aspiration of mediastinal lymph nodes made the use of PET in the evaluation of nodal disease unclear.

Recent retrospective studies have called into question the use of PET in staging the mediastinum in esophageal cancer. The largest of these studies, by Keswani and colleagues[19] from Washington University, evaluated 148 patients who underwent esophageal EUS and PET for staging of esophageal cancer. EUS detected locoregional nodal disease by EUS criteria or cytology in 92 patients. PET was positive in only 41 (45%) of 92 of these patients. For celiac nodal disease, PET identified only 2 of 17 patients with node involvement detected by EUS. Among cases in which nodal disease was confirmed by cytology or histology, EUS was significantly more sensitive than PET (86% vs 44%; P<.001). Nodal staging was not affected in any patient by the addition of PET to a complete EUS examination.

It is the authors' practice to obtain esophageal EUS for nodal staging for all patients undergoing preoperative work-up for esophageal cancer. Paraesophageal lymph nodes are more accurately evaluated initially by EUS because intense signal from the primary tumor often interferes with their evaluation on PET. This may not hold true in regards to restaging after induction chemoradiation. Cerfolio and colleagues[20] demonstrated in a prospective study of 48 patients that PET-CT more accurately identifies residual nodal disease after induction therapy compared with CT and EUS.

There are several additional benefits to obtaining PET imaging in esophageal cancer, mentioned briefly next. PET is useful in the initial evaluation of patients with esophageal cancer to evaluate for distant metastatic disease. A UK multicenter prospective study demonstrated an improvement in pretreatment staging with PET-CT compared with CT and EUS alone. This benefit was seen in the identification of distant metastatic disease.[21] There is also a body of literature to suggest that baseline PET scan, particularly the SUVmax of the tumor, may predict patients likely to respond to preoperative chemotherapy[22,23] and may also predict overall survival.[24] PET has also been proved useful in assessing early metabolic response to induction chemotherapy,[25] indicating that it may serve as a useful guide to treatment during induction therapy. Additionally, the decline in SUV from baseline to postchemoradiation PET has been shown to predict pathologic complete response[20] and survival in some studies.[26,27] The authors do obtain PET-CT imaging on most patients with esophageal cancer, although not for the purpose of mediastinal lymph node staging. It is of questionable benefit to obtain PET imaging on patients with the earliest T1 tumors (ie, the tumors that are detected on asymptomatic patients with flat lesions arising from Barrett esophagus). The prevalence of nodal and distant metastatic disease is likely so low in these patients that the value of the additional staging is negligible.

SUMMARY

FDG-PET and PET-CT imaging have become commonly used modalities in the staging of NSCLC and esophageal cancer. PET is the most accurate noninvasive approach to staging mediastinal lymph nodes in NSCLC. It is valuable in its ability to select patients in whom primary surgical therapy is not optimal by identifying occult N2 nodal disease. PET abnormalities should be confirmed histologically and invasive mediastinal staging should be pursued when the clinical suspicion of N2 disease is high, despite negative PET. The role of PET in mediastinal lymph node staging in esophageal cancer is less clear, having been largely supplanted by EUS. PET remains an important part of the esophageal staging algorithm, although not for its use in identifying nodal

metastases. Perhaps its greatest value in esophageal cancer is the ability to detect distant metastatic disease in patients with larger tumors and known or suspected nodal metastases.

REFERENCES

1. Silvestri G, Gould M, Marolis M, et al. Noninvasive staging of non-small cell lung cancer: ACCP evidence-based clinical practice guidelines (2nd edition). Chest 2007;132:178S–201S.
2. van Tinteren H, Hoekstra O, Smit E, et al. Effectiveness of positron emission tomography in the preoperative assessment of patients with suspected non-small-cell lung cancer: the PLUS multicentre randomised trial. Lancet 2002;359:1388–92.
3. Reed C, Harpole D, Posther K, et al. Results of the American College of Surgeons Oncology Group Z0050 Trial: the utility of positron emission tomography in staging potentially operable non-small cell lung cancer. J Thorac Cardiovasc Surg 2003;126: 1943–51.
4. Viney R, Boyer M, King M, et al. Randomized controlled trial of the role of positron emission tomography in the management of stage I and II non-small cell lung cancer. J Clin Oncol 2004;22: 2357–62.
5. Beyer T, Townsend DW, Brun T, et al. A combined PET/CT scanner for clinical oncology. J Nucl Med 2000;10(Suppl 3):S377–80.
6. Lardinois D, Weder W, Hany T, et al. Staging of non-small-cell lung cancer with integrated positron-emission tomography and computed tomography. N Engl J Med 2003;348:2500–7.
7. Cerfolio RJ, Ojha B, Bryant AS, et al. The accuracy of integrated PET-CT compared with dedicated PET alone for the staging of patients with non-small cell lung cancer. Ann Thorac Surg 2004;78:1017–23.
8. Fischer B, Lassen U, Mortensen J, et al. Preoperative staging of lung cancer with combined PET-CT. N Engl J Med 2009;361:32–9.
9. Maziak D, Darling G, Inculet R, et al. Positron emission tomography in staging early lung cancer: a randomized trial. Ann Intern Med 2009;151:221–8.
10. Darling G, Maziak D, Inculet R, et al. Positron emission tomography-computed tomography compared with invasive mediastinal staging in non-small cell lung cancer: results of mediastinal staging in the early lung positron emission tomography trial. J Thorac Oncol 2011;6:1367–72.
11. Flanagan FL, Dehdashti F, Siegel BA, et al. Staging of esophageal cancer with 18F-flourodeoxyglucose positron emission tomography. Am J Roentgenol 1997;168:417–24.
12. Block MI, Patterson GA, Sundaresan RS, et al. Improvement in staging of esophageal cancer with

the addition of positron emission tomography. Ann Thorac Surg 1997;64:770–6 [discussion: 776–7].

13. Luketich J, Schauer P, Meltzer C, et al. Role of positron emission tomography in staging esophageal cancer. Ann Thorac Surg 1997;64:765–9.

14. van Westreenen H, Westerterp M, Bossuyt P, et al. Systematic review of the staging performance of 18F-flourodeoxyglucose positron emission tomography in esophageal cancer. J Clin Oncol 2004;22:3805–12.

15. Meyers B, Downey R, Decker P, et al. The utility of positron emission tomography in staging of potentially operable carcinoma of the thoracic esophagus: results of the American College of Surgeons Oncology Group Z0060 trial. J Thorac Cardiovasc Surg 2007;133:738–45.

16. Okada M, Murakami T, Kumano S, et al. Integrated FDG-PET/CT compared with intravenous contrast-enhanced CT for evaluation of metastatic regional lymph nods in patients with resectable early stage esophageal cancer. Ann Nucl Med 2009;23:73–80.

17. Schreurs L, Pultrum B, Koopmans K, et al. Better assessment of nodal metastases by PET/CT fusion compared to side-by-side PET/CT in oesophageal cancer. Anticancer Res 2008;28:1867–74.

18. Kato H, Kimura H, Nakajima M, et al. The additional value of integrated PET/CT over PET in initial lymph node staging of esophageal cancer. Oncol Rep 2008;20:857–62.

19. Keswani R, Early D, Edmundowicz S, et al. Routine positron emission tomography does not alter nodal staging in patients undergoing EUS-guided FNA for esophageal cancer. Gastrointest Endosc 2009; 69:1210–7.

20. Cerfolio R, Bryant A, Ohja B, et al. The accuracy of endoscopic ultrasonography with fine-needle aspiration, integrated positron emission tomography with computed tomography, and computed tomography in restaging patients with esophageal cancer after neoadjuvant chemoradiotherapy. J Thorac Cardiovasc Surg 2005;129:1232–41.

21. Noble F, Bailey D. SWCIS Upper Gastrointestinal Tumour Panel. Impact of PET/CT in the staging of oesophageal cancer: a UK population-based cohort study. Clin Radiol 2009;64:699–705.

22. Downey R, Akhurst T, Ilson D, et al. Whole body FDG-PET and the response of esophageal cancer to induction therapy: results of a prospective trial. J Clin Oncol 2003;21:428–32.

23. Rizk N, Tang L, Adusummilli P, et al. Predictive value of initial PET-SUV$_{max}$ in patients with locally advanced esophageal and gastroesophageal junction adenocarcinoma. J Thorac Oncol 2009;4:875–9.

24. Hong D, Lunagomez S, Kim E, et al. Value of baseline positron emission tomography for predicting overall survival in patients with nonmetastatic esophageal or gastroesophageal junction carcinoma. Cancer 2005;104(8):1620–6.

25. Lordick F, Ott K, Krause BJ, et al. PET to assess early metabolic response and to guide treatment of adenocarcinoma of the oesophagogastric junction: the MUNICON phase II trial. Lancet Oncol 2007;8: 797–805.

26. Javeri H, Xiao L, Rohren E, et al. The higher the decrease in the standardized uptake value of positron emission tomography after chemoradiation, the better the survival of patients with gastroesophageal adenocarcinoma. Cancer 2009;115:5184–92.

27. Murthy S, Patnana S, Xiao L, et al. The standardized uptake value of 18-fluorodeoxyglucose positron emission tomography after chemoradiation and clinical outcome in patients with localized gastroesophageal carcinoma. Oncology 2010;78:316–22.

MicroRNAs and Lymph Node Metastatic Disease in Lung Cancer

Francesco Fazi, PhD[a],*, Giulia Fontemaggi, PhD[b]

KEYWORDS

• MicroRNAs • Lymph node metastasis • Lung cancer

Metastatic spread is the most important prognostic factor in patients with lung cancer[1]; it usually occurs through the vascular and lymphatic systems. Cancer cells may use these systems through expression of soluble mediators that can alter the normal pattern of angiogenesis and lymphangiogenesis, leading to the creation of channels for tumor metastasis.[2,3] In early lung cancer the most important mechanism for the spread of tumor is dissemination through the lymphatic system. The propensity to disseminate through either the blood or lymphatic vessels may depend mostly on physical restrictions imposed on invasive tumors, although active mechanisms for attracting cells to specific types of vasculature have also recently emerged. The lymphatic capillaries are relatively large, thin-walled vessels composed of a single layer of endothelial cells. These capillaries are not sheathed by pericytes or smooth muscle cells, and have little or no basement membrane.[4] This configuration inevitably keeps lymphatics "leaky" in comparison with blood vessels, thus lowering the barriers for tumor invasion. In addition, survival of tumor cells may benefit from the passive, low-shear system of fluid transport characteristic of lymphatics. The type of cell movement depends largely on the surrounding extracellular matrix (ECM) and the integrity of cell-to-cell junctions. A fibroblast-like, single-cell migration tends to occur when mature, integrin-containing focal contacts

develop in the presence of dense matrix networks. In the presence of less adhesive conditions, amoeboid migration is instead favored; this can be observed in vivo or in 3-dimensional cultures when focal contacts are lacking.[5] The speed of amoeboid migration is about 10 to 30 times faster than mesenchymal migration and is protease independent. The lymphatic vessels lack basement membranes, and the ECM network is less dense around peritumoral lymphatics than around intratumoral blood vessels; this would allow both the amoeboid-type and the mesenchymal-type intravasation into the lymphatic circulation. Lymphatic permeability may also allow passage of cell aggregates that have retained expression of homotypic cell-to-cell adhesion receptors such as cadherins. In animal models, 0.01% or fewer of the cancer cells entering the circulation develop into metastases.[6,7] Despite this, metastatic spread is common. The sequence of events underlying the metastatic process reflects a series of chromosomal rearrangements in tumor cells as well as changes in the expression of several genes. Among the latter, microRNAs (miRNAs) are emerging as crucial molecules that control the metastatic potential of cancer cells. This review focuses on recent discoveries concerning the involvement of miRNAs in tumorigenesis of lung cancer, with particular emphasis on: (1) the dysregulation of miRNA expression in lung cancer tissue compared

This work was supported by Grants from AIRC (Italian Association for Cancer Research) to F.F. and G.F. The authors have no related disclosures.

[a] Department of Medico-Surgical Sciences and Biotechnologies, Sapienza University of Rome, Corso della Repubblica 79, 04100 Latina, Italy
[b] Translational Oncogenomics Unit, Regina Elena Cancer Institute, Via Elio Chianesi 53, 00144 Rome, Italy
* Corresponding author.
E-mail address: francesco.fazi@uniroma1.it

with normal tissue counterparts; (2) the ability in lung cancer of miRNAs with altered expression and/or hypermethylated miRNAs to predict lymph node positivity.

MICRORNA BIOGENESIS

During normal development an appropriate pattern of epigenetic modifications, including genomic DNA methylation, histone modifications, nucleosome positioning, and expression of small regulatory RNAs contribute to the regulation of gene expression and determination of cell type and tissue specificity. Deregulation of these epigenetic mechanisms results in the establishment of an abnormal cancer epigenome and cooperates with genetic alterations in the development and progression of neoplastic phenotype.[8,9]

miRNAs are a newly described class of small (approximately 22 nucleotides long) noncoding RNAs that function as endogenous posttranscriptional silencers, degrading mRNA and/or impairing translation of specific target genes.[10–13] Of note, miRNA expression is tissue specific and highly regulated according to the cells' developmental lineage and stage, and are involved in the regulation of several physiologic cellular processes including apoptosis, hematopoietic differentiation, metabolism, skin morphogenesis, and neural development.[14–18] Most miRNAs are independent transcriptional units, although many mammalian miRNAs are encoded within intron/exon sequences of protein-coding genes. These miRNAs are transcribed by RNA polymerase II as a long primary miRNA transcript (pri-miRNA), which is then processed into a stem-loop precursor (pre-miRNA) of approximately 70 nucleotides, through the activity of the RNase III endonuclease Drosha and its partner Parsha. Pre-miRNA molecules, in association with the Ran-GTP–dependent factor exportin-5, are actively transported into the cytoplasm where they are processed by the Dicer RNaseIII enzyme into mature 22-nucleotide-long double-stranded miRNA. Subsequent loading of the functional strand of the duplex into the RNA-induced silencing complex (RISC) enables the miRNA to recognize its target messenger RNA; miRNAs recognize their target mRNAs mainly through limited base-pairing interaction between the 5'-end "seed" region (2–8 nucleotides from the 5'-end) and the complementary sequences in the 3'-untranslated regions (3'-UTRs) of phylogenetically conserved target mRNAs. Just few animal miRNAs have sufficient complementarities to mRNAs that allow their cleavage ("slicing"). The majority of the animal miRNAs imprecisely match

their targets, resulting in target mRNAs destabilization by nonslicer mechanisms, including inhibition of translation initiation or elongation, premature termination of translation (ribosome drop-off), deadenylation, and other forms of translational repression (ie, decapping). After being targeted by miRNAs, mRNAs can also undergo concentration, exclusion from translational machinery, degradation, or storage in large, macroscopic, cytoplasmic foci, named processing bodies (p-bodies). The p-bodies contain a wide range of enzymes involved in RNA turnover, including decapping enzymes, deadenylases, and exonucleases.[19]

The deregulation of miRNA expression has been related to human developmental defects and tumor progression since several miRNAs were identified as a new class of genes with tumor-suppressor and oncogenic functions.[20–24] The localization of nonrandom chromosomal abnormalities or other types of genetic alterations and the establishment of an abnormal cancer epigenome at miRNA genomic regions (observed in several cancer phenotypes) strongly underline the contribution of the deregulation of miRNA expression to the malignancy process.[25]

Advances in expression technologies have facilitated the high-throughput analysis of small RNAs, identifying novel miRNAs and showing unique miRNA signatures specifically associated with normal or tumor-derived samples.[26–28] Hence, a new molecular taxonomy of human cancers based on miRNA expression profiling has been proposed. Indeed it was recently found that miRNA profiles are more informative than messenger RNA profiles, and could classify poorly differentiated tumors because they better reflect the developmental lineage and differentiation state of cancer.[29] To date, unique miRNA signatures have been identified as new molecular markers relevant to the pathogenesis, diagnosis, and prognosis in several malignant tumors, including lung, neuroblastoma, colon, pancreatic, and leukemic.[28,29]

MICRORNAs ALTERED IN LUNG CANCER: ONCOGENES AND TUMOR SUPPRESSORS

As already mentioned, the expression of specific subsets of miRNAs can be altered in lung cancer, as in other cancers (**Table 1**). Much experimental evidence now assigns specific functions to those miRNAs that are overexpressed or underexpressed in transformed cells. The majority of the studies are based on the reintroduction of downregulated miRNAs or on the inhibition of upregulated miRNAs in cancer cell lines, followed by the

Table 1
Examples of relevant microRNAs in lung cancer

MicroRNA	Comment	Expression	References
let7 family	Tumor suppressor activity	↓NSCLC, ↓SCC	30–32,36,37
miR-17-92 cluster	Oncogenic properties	↑SCLC, ↑SCC	33,36
miR-31	Oncogenic properties	↑Lung cancer	34
miR-146b	Prognostic	↑SCC	36
miR-21	Oncogenic properties High serum levels associated with LN+	↑SCC NSCLC	35,37,50,51
miR-155	Prognostic	↑SCC, ↑AC	36,37,55–57
Signature: high (miR-145, miR-17-3p, miR-106, miR-93, miR-155, miR-21), low (let-7a-2, let-7b or miR-145)	Unfavorable prognosis	NSCLC	37
miR-200c	Epithelial-mesenchymal transition	↓NSCLC	40
miR-451	Predictor of LN+	↓NSCLC	52
miR-130a	Predictor of LN+	↑NSCLC	53
miR-125a	Predictor of LN+	↓NSCLC	54
miR-148, miR-34b/c, miR-9	Hypermethylation associated with LN+	↓NSCLC	60,61
Signature: high (miR-142-5p, miR-148a and 148b, miR-369-3p, miR-215, miR-152, miR-155), low (miR-373, miR-138-1)	Differentially expressed between primary tumors and the related lymph node metastasis	Lung cancer	62

Abbreviations: LN+, lymph node positivity; NSCLC, non–small cell lung cancer; SCC, squamous cell carcinoma; SCLC, small cell lung cancer.

assessment of the phenotypic changes occurring in the cells as well as the characterization of the molecular pathways affected.

The let-7 family is a group of miRNAs whose gene sequences mapped to different chromosomal regions are frequently altered in lung cancer. Studies in non–small cell lung cancer (NSCLC) cell lines showed that the induction of high levels of expression of miRNA let-7 inhibits tumor growth and reduces cell-cycle progression. In animal models, the ectopic expression of let-7 reduces the tumor mass and the formation of lung adeno-carcinomas; the reduced expression of let-7 in patients with NSCLC correlates with a poor prognosis. Such experimental and clinical evidence, in addition to negative regulation by the miRNA let-7 of several oncogenes, including RAS, MYC, HMGA2, and several regulators of cell-cycle progression such as cyclin D2, CDK6, and CDC25A, suggest that members belonging to this family of miRNAs play key roles as tumor suppressors in the pathogenesis of lung cancer.[30–32]

Contrarily to the let-7 family of miRNA, all members of the cluster miR-17-92 (miR-17, miR-18a, miR-19a, miR-20a, miR-19b-1, and miR-92-1) are considered oncogenes.[33] These miRNAs cooperate with c-Myc in accelerating tumor development and in promoting tumor neovascularization. The miRNAs of this cluster are expressed at high levels in small lung cancer cells and promote tumorigenesis through the inactivation of the reti-noblastoma (RB) protein. The molecular identification of the role of these miRNAs in the onset of cancer provides the possibility of using these small RNAs as potential molecular targets for the development of treatment protocols increasingly targeted at and considered effective for the treatment of small cell lung cancer.

miR-31 is another example of miRNA with onco-genic properties in lung cancer.[34] Inactivation in vivo of miR-31 causes a reduction in tumor clonal growth and tumor aggressiveness. The oncogenic activity of miR-31 is closely linked to its ability to directly suppress tumor suppressors; this regulatory circuit is crucial for the control of cell proliferation in lung cancer.

In vivo studies have recently shown that increased expression of miR-21 causes an effective reduction of apoptosis in NSCLC. Using mice transgenic for the loss or gain of function of miR-21, Hatley and colleagues[35] found that the increased expression of miR-21 results in an increase in tumorigenesis and, conversely, its genetic deletion partially protects from tumor formation. The expression of miR-21 increases as a result of oncogenic k-Ras activity and is able to modulate the tumorigenicity of NSCLC; it regulates negatively the signaling pathway of Ras/MEK/ERK, important for the induction the apoptotic process. It was also shown that miR-21 deletion significantly sensitizes to chemotherapy treatment with DNA-damaging agents, suggesting that inhibition of miR-21 may also play a major role in chemotherapy planning for NSCLC.[35]

Besides the functional characterization of single miRNAs with altered expression in lung cancer cells, an additional research strategy emerged in the last years aiming to identify miRNA changes in lung cancer tissues from a global point of view. These genome-wide studies have identified groups (signatures) of miRNAs with altered expression between primary cancer samples and the corresponding noncancerous tissues; they have also showed that these signatures may be extremely important in terms of diagnostic, predictive, and prognostic power. The fact that miRNAs are well preserved in formalin-fixed paraffin-embedded tissues also makes them attractive and promising candidates for use in routinely processed material.

A study performed by Raponi and colleagues[36] evaluated the different expression of miRNAs between 61 squamous cell lung cancer (SCC) specimens and 10 matched normal lung samples. A molecular signature comprising 15 miRNAs distinguishing SCC from normal lung was identified, including members of the miR-17-92 cluster and its paralogues. Some of the identified miRNAs such as miR-155 and let-7 were previously shown to have prognostic value in adenocarcinoma. Among these miRNAs the differential expression of miR-146b showed the strongest predictive accuracy for stratifying prognostic groups, at approximately 78%.

A previous study by Yanaihara and colleagues[37] evaluated the predictive power of miRNAs, showing different expression levels in tumor specimens from a cohort of patients with lung cancer. In this study no normal matched controls were analyzed. A prognostic power for a subset of miRNA was identified. It was shown that patients with high expression of either miR-155, miR-17-3p, miR-106a, miR-93, or mir-21 and low expression of either let-7a-2, let-7b, or miR-145 had an unfavorable prognosis.

These results indicate that miRNA expression profiles represent a potential diagnostic and prognostic tool for the management of lung cancer.

ROLE OF MICRORNAs IN METASTATIC PROGRESSION

A growing list of reports suggests that miRNAs could play a crucial role not only in tumor growth, carcinogenesis, and response to chemotherapy but also in the metastatic progression of different malignancies. Metastasis is a complex, multistep process by which primary tumor cells invade adjacent tissue, enter the systemic circulation, and finally proliferate with secondary lesions.

A primary process for the development of metastases is the so-called epithelial-mesenchymal transition (EMT). The EMT is an extremely common event during embryonic development whereas it is very rare in adult human cells, where it is found mostly during wound healing and fibrosis of the kidney. During EMT, epithelial cells lose cell-to-cell contact, mainly mediated by the adhesion molecule E-cadherin, and undergo cytoskeletal remodeling and changes in cell polarity, resulting in the acquisition of a mesenchymal morphology and an increase in cell motility. Tumor cells exploit these characteristics to acquire invasive capacity. In fact, the conversion to a mesenchymal stage allows the tumor epithelial cells to detach from the primary tumor, invade the basement membrane, enter the bloodstream, and colonize distal tissues. The EMT is a reversible process and tumor cells, once the target tissue is colonized, regain a proliferative epithelial phenotype by promoting the formation and development of a polarized epithelium in secondary metastatic sites. Various miRNAs involved in the negative regulation of EMT and metastatic process have been identified recently. For example, the miRNAs belonging to the family of miR-200 (miR-200a, miR-200b, miR-200c, miR-141, and miR-429) were recently identified as powerful modulators of EMT. These miRNAs cooperatively regulate the expression of the transcriptional repressors ZEB1 and ZEB2, which are responsible for the transcriptional repression of the gene-encoding E-cadherin.[38,39] The induction of ectopic miR-200 family members results in an increased expression of E-cadherin and a reduction of the motility of cancer cells. Conversely, inhibition of the expression of miR-200 induces EMT in tumor cell lines expressing high basal levels of these miRNAs. Studies in mouse models of lung adenocarcinoma have further confirmed the involvement of miR-200 family members in the regulation of EMT and in the modulation of pulmonary metastatic potential of tumor cells.[40] The expression of miR-200c was investigated in a panel of NSCLC cell lines, and a strong inverse correlation with invasion was detected. Reintroduction of miR-200c into highly invasive/aggressive NSCLC cells induced a loss of the mesenchymal phenotype by restoring E-cadherin and reducing N-cadherin expression, and inhibited in vitro cell invasion as well as metastatic spread in vivo. In tumor specimens obtained from 69 consecutive patients undergoing NSCLC resection, lower levels of miR-200c expression were found to be associated with a poor grade of differentiation ($P = .04$), a higher propensity toward lymphatic spread ($P<.01$), and a lower E-cadherin expression ($P = .01$). These data indicate that the loss of miR-200c expression induces an aggressive, invasive, and chemoresistant phenotype, and that assessment of its expression could contribute toward improving the clinicopathologic definition of patients with NSCLC.[40]

MICRORNA INVOLVEMENT IN LYMPH NODE METASTASIS IN LUNG CANCER

Distant metastasis is responsible for 90% of deaths in patients with solid tumors, and the status of regional lymph nodes is crucial for staging, treatment planning, and evaluation of results in patients with lung cancer. The lymphatic route of metastasis is particularly relevant for carcinomas, where regional lymph nodes are often the first organs to develop metastasis and might serve as a potential "bridgehead" in further dissemination.[41,42] Micrometastasis to lymph nodes is thought to occur in most primary tumors before they are clinically detectable, and therefore can be the most significant prognostic indicator in many human cancers.[43] Occult lymph node metastases (undetected by conventional methods) have been seen in up to 20% of T1 and T2 lung cancer tumors.[44,45] Positive emission tomography (PET) has demonstrated more sensitivity and specificity than computed tomography for mediastinal lymph node assessment in patients with potentially operable NSCLC.[46] However, PET might underestimate micrometastases, and especially microscopic nodal disease, due to its limitation for detection of lesions smaller than 4 to 5 mm.[47,48] PET cannot detect small metastases or micrometastases because of the lower limits of resolution of the PET camera. The identification of molecular biomarkers whose expression in the surgically resected tumor tissue or in patients' serum and plasma is able to accurately assess the presence of micrometastases is strongly needed. Some examples of promising miRNAs recently identified are given in **Table 1**.

MICRORNA EXPRESSION AS A PREDICTIVE MARKER FOR LYMPH NODE METASTASIS

miRNAs have recently been identified in serum and plasma, in a remarkably stable form that is protected from endogenous RNase activity. Several publications have reported on the deregulation of circulating miRNAs in the blood of tumor patients,[49] but there are only a few reports on circulating miRNAs in serum or plasma of NSCLC patients. Two studies have very recently reported that miR-21 is expressed at higher levels in serum from NSCLC patients when compared with control samples. High serum miR-21 was significantly correlated with lymph node metastasis and advanced clinical stage of NSCLC patients. In these studies miR-21 expression in serum behaves as an independent prognostic factor.[50,51] These studies indicate that miR-21 may be a potential biomarker for the diagnosis and prognosis of NSCLC patients.

In addition to circulating miRNAs in plasma and serum, the expression of specific miRNAs in the tumor specimen is also being attributed increasing relevance for its ability to act as a predictive biomarker for lymph node positivity as well as for other clinicopathological features. For example Wang and colleagues,[52] by comparing miRNA expression profiling of NSCLC tissues with that of corresponding nontumor lung tissues, observed that miR-451 is significantly downregulated in NSCLC and that a decreased miR-451 expression correlates with lymph node metastasis. This molecular marker was also associated with poor tumor differentiation, advanced pathologic stage, and poor prognosis.

An additional miRNA found to be deregulated and associated with lymph node status in lung cancer is miR-130a. Wang and colleagues[53] observed that miR-130a expression is indeed increased in NSCLC. The statistical analysis showed that overexpression of miR-130a was strongly associated with lymph node metastasis, staging, and poor prognosis. Moreover, there was a significant difference in miR-130a expression levels between smokers and nonsmokers. Multivariate Cox regression analysis showed that miR-130a was an independent prognostic factor in patients with NSCLC.

At the molecular level, miR-130a has been shown to play a role in antagonizing the inhibitory effects of GAX on endothelial cell proliferation, migration, and tube formation, and in antagonizing the inhibitory effects of HoxA5 on tube formation in vitro, which means that NSCLC overexpressing miR-130a probably more efficiently induces neo-angiogenesis. These data suggest that miR-130a may represent a potential novel prognostic marker for NSCLC.[53]

Jiang and colleagues[54] demonstrated changes in the expression of 2 miRNAs that are generated from the maturation of pre–miR-125a, named miR-125a-3p and miR-125a-5p. miR-125a-5p down-modulation in NSCLC was previously reported also by Yanaihara and colleagues.[37] In this subsequent study pre-miR-125a–derived mature miR-NAs were analyzed by quantitative reverse transcription–polymerase chain reaction (RT-PCR) in 52 matched NSCLC specimens and in adjacent tissues. Expression of both miR-125a-5p and miR-125a-3p was decreased significantly in NSCLC. Furthermore, the results from the Spearman correlation test showed a negative relationship between hsa-miR-125a-3p expression and pathologic stage or lymph node metastasis, and an inverse relationship between hsa-miR-125a-5p expression and pathologic stage or lymph node metastasis. In vitro gain-of-function experiments indicated that hsa-miR-125a-3p and hsa-miR-125a-5p function in an opposing manner, suppressing or enhancing cell migration and invasion in A549 and SPC-A-1 cell lines, respectively.[54]

Donnem and colleagues[55] presented the first large-scale study combining high-throughput tissue microarrays (TMA) and in situ hybridization to evaluate the prognostic impact of miR-155 expression. miR-155 was previously reported to be overexpressed in NSCLC by several studies.[36,37,56,57] Some of these also showed a prognostic impact of miR-155 expression using quantitative RT-PCR. Most of the previous studies on miRNA expression were done on microarrays using RNA extracted from human cancer specimens and containing a mixture of neoplastic tumor cells and tumor stromal cells. In situ hybridization provides the crucial advantage of being able to identify precisely positive signals at the cellular level, enabling a more accurate characterization of cancer cells. For instance, recent data have demonstrated that some miRNAs show high expression levels in stromal cells but not in tumor cells.[58] The use of in situ hybridization avoids artifacts based on tumor cell composition. In an unselected population of surgically resected NSCLC (comprising 191 SCCs, 95 adenocarcinomas [ACs], 31 large cell carcinomas, and 18 bronchioalveolar carcinomas), high miR-155 expression was an independent negative prognostic factor in AC, whereas high miR-155 expression was an independent favorable prognosticator in SCC with regional nodal metastasis. These findings indicate that each miRNA could even exert opposite functions, depending on the histologic type and the stage of the disease.[55]

HYPERMETHYLATION OF SPECIFIC MICRORNA GENOMIC LOCI AS A PREDICTIVE MARKER FOR LYMPH NODE METASTASIS

As extensively reported previously, miRNAs can be downregulated in cancer. As for classic metastasis suppressor genes, whose promoter CpG island hypermethylation leads to expression silencing, miRNAs with tumor-suppressor features also can present methylation-associated silencing in human cancers.[59] To unmask hypermethylated miRNAs that contribute in vivo and in vitro to the formation of lymph node metastasis, Esteller's group[60] performed miRNA expression microarray analysis on DNA-demethylating drug treatment in cancer cells. Through this approach they identified CpG island hypermethylation of miR-148, miR-34b/c, and the miR-9 family. These results were confirmed on a group of primary tumor samples, including colon, lung, breast, head, and neck cancer, and melanoma. When miRNA hypermethylation was evaluated with respect to the existence or not of lymph node metastasis, the presence of miR-34b/c, miR-148, and miR-9-3 CpG island hypermethylation in the primary tumor (lung, breast, melanoma) was significantly associated with those tumors that were positive for metastatic cancer cells in the corresponding lymph nodes, which highlights the importance of the in vivo role of miRNA epigenetic silencing in metastasis formation. miR-34b hypermethylation was also very recently observed by Watanabe and colleagues[61] in 41% of 99 primary NSCLC analyzed. Also in this study, the DNA methylation of miR-34b was significantly associated with lymphatic invasion. These results suggest that miRNA methylation may be used in clinical practice as a marker to predict tumor prognosis and metastatic behavior. Most importantly, this could also provide the molecular basis for a new therapeutic use for pharmacologic compounds with DNA-demethylating activity in the treatment of cancer patients with metastatic disease.

MICRORNAs ARE DIFFERENTIALLY EXPRESSED BETWEEN PRIMARY TUMORS AND METASTATIC LYMPH NODES

miRNAs are frequently altered in their expression in the tumor in comparison with the normal adjacent tissue. Given that only few cells are fully metastatic in the primary tumor, it is expected that molecular alterations characterizing the entire tumor mass are not the major factor responsible for metastasis. Many efforts are actually aimed at identifying molecular alterations that enable the metastatic process, and one of the more promising approaches is the analysis of differences in the expression profiles of matched primary versus metastatic tumors.

To seek a specific miRNA expression signature characterizing the metastatic phenotype of solid tumors, an miRNA microarray analysis on 43 paired primary tumors (colon, bladder, breast, and lung cancers) and one of their related metastatic lymph nodes was performed.[62] In this study a metastatic cancer miRNA signature comprising 15 overexpressed and 17 underexpressed miRNAs was demonstrated. These results were also confirmed by quantitative RT-PCR analysis. Some of the identified miRNAs show a well-characterized association with cancer progression (eg, miR-10b, miR-21, miR-30a, miR-30e, miR-125b, miR-141, miR-200b, miR-200c, and miR-205). miRNAs that were able to differentiate between primary tumors and the related metastatic samples by specific organ of origin were also identified in this study. No statistically significant overlap was found between the signatures for specific organs and those for the group of tumors as a whole. Lung-specific signatures included miR-142-5p, miR-148a, miR-148b, miR-369-3p, miR-215, miR-152, and miR-155 (upregulated), as well as miR-373 and miR-138-1 (downregulated).

SUMMARY

The classification of lung cancer based on histologic type and nodal status is the most important determinant in planning treatment strategy. However, a considerable variability in prognosis has been observed for subsets of patients with the same clinical features. Consequently, the clinical incorporation of predictive and prognostic molecular biomarkers with traditional cancer staging should improve the management of patients with lung cancer, leading to stratification of patients sharing signatures of molecular markers. miRNAs are among the most promising biomarkers that will be probably incorporated soon into clinical practice. The alteration of the expression of these molecules as well as their epigenetic modulation in cancer represents molecular features strongly associated with the metastatic behavior of cancer cells and with lymph node involvement. These observations indicate that miRNAs represent promising tools for the prognosis of lung cancer and, more importantly, for the development of novel therapeutic strategies aimed at interfering with the metastatic potential of cancer cells.

REFERENCES

1. Pepper MS. Lymphangiogenesis and tumor metastasis: myth or reality? Clin Cancer Res 2001;7: 462–8.
2. Shayan R, Achen MG, Stacker SA. Lymphatic vessels in cancer metastasis: bridging gaps. Carcinogenesis 2006;27:1729–38.
3. Alitalo K, Tammela T, Petrova TV. Lymphangiogenesis in development and human disease. Nature 2005;438:946–53.
4. Alitalo K, Carmeliet P. Molecular mechanisms of lymphangiogenesis in health and disease. Cancer Cell 2002;1:219–27.
5. Sahai E, Marshall CJ. Differing modes of tumour cell invasion have distinct requirements for Rho/ROCK signaling and extracellular proteolysis. Nat Cell Biol 2003;5:711–8.
6. Chambers AF, Groom AC, MacDonald IC. Dissemination and growth of cancer cells in metastatic sites. Nat Rev Cancer 2002;2:563–72.
7. Luzzi KJ, MacDonald IC, Schmidt EE, et al. Multistep nature of metastatic inefficiency: dormancy of solitary cells after successful extravasation and limited survival of early micrometastases. Am J Pathol 1998;153:865–73.
8. Kumar MS, Lu J, Mercer KL, et al. Impaired microRNA processing enhances cellular transformation and tumorigenesis. Nat Genet 2007;39:673–7.
9. Egger G, Liang G, Aparicio A, et al. Epigenetics in human disease and prospects for epigenetic therapy. Nature 2004;429:457–63.
10. Ambros V. The functions of animal microRNAs. Nature 2004;431:350–5.
11. He L, Hannon GJ. MicroRNAs: small RNAs with a big role in gene regulation. Nat Rev Genet 2004; 5(7):522–31.
12. Bartel DP. MicroRNAs: target recognition and regulatory functions. Cell 2009;136:215–33.
13. Krol J, Loedige I, Filipowicz W. The widespread regulation of microRNA biogenesis, function and decay. Nat Rev Genet 2010;11:597–610.
14. Chen CZ, Li L, Lodish HF, et al. MicroRNAs modulate hematopoietic lineage differentiation. Science 2004;303:83–6.
15. Poy MN, Eliasson L, Krutzfeldt J, et al. A pancreatic islet-specific microRNA regulates insulin secretion. Nature 2004;432:226–30.
16. Yi R, O'Carroll D, Pasolli HA, et al. Morphogenesis in skin is governed by discrete sets of differentially expressed microRNAs. Nat Genet 2006;38:356–62.
17. Kosik KS. The neuronal microRNA system. Nat Rev Neurosci 2006;7:911–20.

18. Fazi F, Nervi C. MicroRNA: basic mechanisms and transcriptional regulatory networks for cell fate determination. Cardiovasc Res 2008;79:553–61.

19. Eulalio A, Behm-Ansmant I, Izaurralde E. P bodies: at the crossroads of post-transcriptional pathways. Nat Rev Mol Cell Biol 2007;8(1):9–22.

20. Mendell JT. MicroRNAs: critical regulators of development, cellular physiology and malignancy. Cell Cycle 2005;4:1179–84.

21. He L, Thomson JM, Hemann MT, et al. A microRNA polycistron as a potential human oncogene. Nature 2005;435:828–33.

22. Kent OA, Mendell JT. A small piece in the cancer puzzle: microRNA as tumor suppressors and oncogene. Oncogene 2006;25:6188–96.

23. Hummond SM. MicroRNA as oncogenes. Curr Opin Genet Dev 2006;16:4–9.

24. Esequela-Kercher A, Slack FJ. Oncomir—microRNA with a role in cancer. Nat Rev Cancer 2006;6:259–69.

25. Deng S, Calin GA, Croce CM, et al. Mechanisms of microRNA deregulation in human cancer. Cell Cycle 2008;7(17):2643–6.

26. Lu J, Getz G, Miska EA, et al. MicroRNA expression profiles classify human cancer. Nature 2005;435: 834–8.

27. Calin GA, Ferracin M, Cimmino A, et al. A microRNA signature associated with prognosis and progression in chronic lymphocytic leukaemia. N Engl J Med 2005;353:1793–801.

28. Cummins JM, Velculescu VE. Implication of microRNA profiling for cancer diagnosis. Oncogene 2006;25:6220–7.

29. Cortez MA, Ivan C, Zhou P, et al. MicroRNAs in cancer: from bench to bedside. Adv Cancer Res 2010;108:113–57.

30. Takamizawa J, Konishi H, Yanagisawa K, et al. Reduced expression of the let-7 microRNAs in human lung cancers in association with shortened postoperative survival. Cancer Res 2004;64(11): 3753–6.

31. Mayr C, Hemann MT, Bartel DP. Disrupting the pairing between let-7 and HMGA2 enhances oncogenic transformation. Science 2007;315:1576–9.

32. Kumar MS, Erkeland SJ, Pester RE, et al. Suppression of non-small cell lung tumor development by the let-7 microRNA family. Proc Natl Acad Sci U S A 2008;105(10):3903–8.

33. Mendell JT. miRiad roles for the miR-17-92 cluster in development and disease. Cell 2008;133:217–22.

34. Liu X, Sempere LF, Ouyang H, et al. MicroRNA-31 functions as an oncogenic microRNA in mouse and human lung cancer cells by repressing specific tumor suppressors. J Clin Invest 2010; 120(4):1298–309.

35. Hatley ME, Patrick DM, Garcia MR, et al. Modulation of K-Ras-dependent lung tumorigenesis by MicroRNA-21. Cancer Cell 2010;18(3):282–93.

36. Raponi M, Dossey L, Jatkoe T, et al. MicroRNA classifiers for predicting prognosis of squamous cell lung cancer. Cancer Res 2009;69:5776–83.

37. Yanaihara N, Caplen N, Bowman E, et al. Unique microRNA molecular profiles in lung cancer diagnosis and prognosis. Cancer Cell 2006;9:189–98.

38. Park SM, Gaur AB, Lengyel E, et al. The miR-200 family determines the epithelial phenotype of cancer cells by targeting the E-cadherin repressors ZEB1 and ZEB2. Genes Dev 2008;22(7):894–907.

39. Gregory PA, Bert AG, Paterson EL, et al. The miR-200 family and miR-205 regulate epithelial to mesenchymal transition by targeting ZEB1 and SIP1. Nat Cell Biol 2008;10(5):593–601.

40. Ceppi P, Mudduluru G, Kumarswamy R, et al. Loss of miR-200c expression induces an aggressive, invasive, and chemoresistant phenotype in non-small cell lung cancer. Mol Cancer Res 2010;8(9): 1207–16.

41. Sleeman JP. The lymph node as a bridgehead in the metastatic dissemination of tumors. Recent Results Cancer Res 2000;157:55–81.

42. Jackson DG. Lymphatic markers, tumour lymphangiogenesis and lymph node metastasis. Cancer Treat Res 2007;135:39–53.

43. Fidler IJ. The pathogenesis of cancer metastasis: the 'seed and soil' hypothesis revisited. Nat Rev Cancer 2003;3:453–8.

44. Asamura H, Suzuki K, Kondo H. Where is the boundary between N1 and N2 station in lung cancer? Ann Thorac Surg 2000;70:1839–45.

45. Wu J, Ohta Y, Minato H, et al. Nodal occult metastasis in patients with peripheral lung adenocarcinoma of 2.0 cm or less in diameter. Ann Thorac Surg 2001;71:1772–8.

46. Pieterman RM, van Putten JW, Meuzelaar JJ, et al. Preoperative staging of non-small cell lung cancer with positron-emission tomography. N Engl J Med 2000;343:254–61.

47. Kernstine KH, Mclaughlin KA, Menda Y, et al. Can FDG-PET reduce the need for mediastinoscopy in potentially resectable non-small cell lung cancer? Ann Thorac Surg 2002;73:394–402.

48. Nomori H, Watanabe K, Ohtsuka T, et al. The size of metastatic foci and lymph node staging yielding false-negative and false-positive lymph node staging with positron emission tomography in patients with lung cancer. J Thorac Cardiovasc Surg 2004;127: 1087–92.

49. Mitchell PS, Parkin RK, Kroh EM, et al. Circulating microRNAs as stable blood-based markers for cancer detection. Proc Natl Acad Sci U S A 2008; 105(30):10513–8.

50. Liu XG, Zhu WY, Huang YY, et al. High expression of serum miR-21 and tumor miR-200c associated with poor prognosis in patients with lung cancer. Med Oncol 2011. [Epub ahead of print].

51. Wang ZX, Bian HB, Wang JR, et al. Prognostic significance of serum miRNA-21 expression in human non-small cell lung cancer. J Surg Oncol 2011;104(7):847–51.
52. Wang R, Wang ZX, Yang JS, et al. MicroRNA-451 functions as a tumor suppressor in human non-small cell lung cancer by targeting ras-related protein 14 (RAB14). Oncogene 2011;30(23):2644–58.
53. Wang XC, Tian LL, Wu HL, et al. Expression of miRNA-130a in non small cell lung cancer. Am J Med Sci 2010;340(5):385–8.
54. Jiang L, Huang Q, Zhang S, et al. Hsa-miR-125a-3p and hsa-miR-125a-5p are downregulated in non-small cell lung cancer and have inverse effects on invasion and migration of lung cancer cells. BMC Cancer 2010;10:318.
55. Donnem T, Eklo K, Berg T, et al. Prognostic impact of MiR-155 in non-small cell lung cancer evaluated by in situ hybridization. J Transl Med 2011;9:6.
56. Volinia S, Calin GA, Liu CG, et al. A microRNA expression signature of human solid tumors defines cancer gene targets. Proc Natl Acad Sci U S A 2006; 103(7):2257–61.
57. Voortman J, Goto A, Mendiboure J, et al. MicroRNA expression and clinical outcomes in patients treated with adjuvant chemotherapy after complete resection of non-small cell lung carcinoma. Cancer Res 2010;70(21):8288–98.
58. Hu Y, Correa AM, Hoque A, et al. Prognostic significance of differentially expressed miRNAs in esophageal cancer. Int J Cancer 2011;128:132–43.
59. Saito Y, Liang G, Egger G, et al. Specific activation of microRNA-127 with downregulation of the proto-oncogene BCL6 by chromatin-modifying drugs in human cancer cells. Cancer Cell 2006;9(6):435–43.
60. Lujambio A, Calin GA, Villanueva A, et al. A microRNA DNA methylation signature for human cancer metastasis. Proc Natl Acad Sci U S A 2008;105(36):13556–61.
61. Watanabe K, Emoto N, Hamano E, et al. Genome structure-based screening identified epigenetically silenced microRNA associated with invasiveness in non-small-cell lung cancer. Int J Cancer 2011. [Epub ahead of print].
62. Baffa R, Fassan M, Volinia S, et al. MicroRNA expression profiling of human metastatic cancers identifies cancer gene targets. J Pathol 2009;219(2):214–21.

Invasive Staging of Mediastinal Lymph Nodes: Mediastinoscopy and Remediastinoscopy

Ramón Rami-Porta, MD, PhD, FETCS*, Sergi Call, MD, FETCS

KEYWORDS
- Lung cancer staging • Mediastinal lymph nodes
- Mediastinoscopy • Remediastinoscopy

Confirmation of nodal status in lung cancer is essential for planning treatment and assessing prognosis. Nodal involvement is associated with poor prognosis. This is especially true for ipsilateral and subcarinal nodal involvement (N2 disease) and for contralateral hilar, mediastinal, and contralateral and ipsilateral supraclavicular nodal involvement (N3 disease). For clinically staged non–small cell lung cancer, 5-year survival rates for N2 and N3 disease are 16% and 7%, respectively. Those for pathologically staged tumors are 22% and 6%, respectively.[1] As for small cell lung cancer, the corresponding rates for clinically staged N2 and N3 tumors are 12% and 9%, respectively,[2] and 6% and 0% for pathologically staged tumors, respectively.[3]

Treatment failures after complete resection of stage III tumors are mainly caused by distant metastasis or by a combination of distant metastasis and locoregional recurrence.[4] To improve survival by controlling subclinical distant metastases, multimodality treatment protocols, including induction chemotherapy followed by lung resection, were introduced in clinical practice. The results of the first published reports showing that induction chemotherapy followed by lung resection was associated with significantly better survival than resection alone[5,6] have been recently confirmed by a meta-analysis of 13 randomized

clinical trials: the hazard ratio for those patients with stage III tumors who received combined therapy was 0.84 (confidence interval, 0.75–0.95).[7] It was generally agreed that the administration of induction therapy had to be based on pathologic evidence of nodal disease, either by transbronchial needle aspiration, by transparietal needle aspiration, or by mediastinoscopy, by far the most used procedure.

More than a decade later, two clinical trials tried to establish the role of resection after induction chemotherapy[8] or chemoradiotherapy[9] for pathologically proved stage III-N2 non–small cell lung cancer. The results of these trials showed that resection did not add any benefit to the whole group of patients. However, subgroup analyses in both trials showed that 5-year survival rates for patients with tumors that had been downstaged from clinical N2 to either pathologic N0 or N1 after induction were significantly higher than those for patients with tumors with persistent mediastinal nodal disease. In one of the studies, 5-year survival rates for pathologic N0-1 and N2 tumors, and for incompletely resected tumors, either with microscopic (R1) or macroscopic (R2) residual disease, were 29%, 7%, and 7% (P = .001), respectively.[8] In the other study, 5-year survival rates for pathologic N0, N1–3, and unresectable tumors were 41%, 24%, and 8% (P = .0001),

The authors have nothing to disclose.
Thoracic Surgery Service, Hospital Universitari Mutua Terrassa, University of Barcelona, Plaza Drive Robert 5, 08221 Terrassa, Barcelona, Spain
* Corresponding author.
E-mail address: rramip@yahoo.es

Thorac Surg Clin 22 (2012) 177–189
doi:10.1016/j.thorsurg.2011.12.003
1547-4127/12/$ – see front matter © 2012 Elsevier Inc. All rights reserved.

respectively.[9] These results showed that resection after induction chemotherapy or chemoradiotherapy cannot be performed indiscriminately. Some selection after induction therapy is necessary, especially the identification of those patients whose tumors have been downstaged from clinical N2 to N0 or N1, because these patients are most likely to benefit from tumor resection. Restaging of these tumors after induction is essential to determine objective tumor response and downstaging. The same methods used for staging can be applied at restaging,[10] but only those providing cytologic or pathologic proof of tumor response and downstaging are reliable enough to make further therapeutic decisions.

In the past decade, less invasive procedures, such as endobronchial ultrasound-guided fine-needle aspiration (EBUS-FNA)[11] and esophageal ultrasound-guided FNA (EUS-FNA)[12] have been progressively introduced in clinical practice. However, more thorough mediastinal explorations have been developed with the objective to remove the upper mediastinal nodes: video-assisted mediastinoscopic lymphadenectomy[13,14] and transcervical extended mediastinal lymphadenectomy.[15] These procedures are described elsewhere in this issue.

Currently, mediastinoscopy and remediastinoscopy must be thoughtfully integrated in clinical practice with all the other procedures that provide cytohistologic evidence of nodal status. They still have an important role in the invasive staging of mediastinal lymph nodes not only in patients with lung cancer, but also in those with mesothelioma and with potentially resectable lung metastases with radiologic or metabolic evidence of mediastinal nodal disease.

MEDIASTINOSCOPY
Historical Note

Mediastinoscopy was first described by Carlens in 1959.[16] Carlens had started mediastinoscopy in 1957 and had performed over 100 procedures without complications by the time he wrote his report. He described the technique and six cases as examples. In cases of suspected or diagnosed lung cancer, he indicated mediastinoscopy if the carina was fixed at rigid bronchoscopy or there was mediastinal widening on chest radiographs. Positive nodes at mediastinoscopy precluded resection. He duly acknowledged his predecessors, Daniels, Harken, and Radner, who also had tried to diagnose intrathoracic diseases without relying to thoracotomy. Daniels described the biopsy of scalene lymph nodes, which could be involved by the same intrathoracic disease and thus avoid exploratory thoracotomy.[17] Harken and colleagues[18] took advantage of the supraclavicular incision used by Daniels to insert a laryngoscope and perform a rudimentary unilateral mediastinoscopy. Radner[19] favored a suprasternal incision to reach paratracheal lymph nodes on both sides. Two of the six cases described by Carlens were for benign diseases: tracheal narrowing and paratracheal cyst. In one of the reported cases, diagnosis of lung cancer was obtained at mediastinoscopy, because there were no endobronchial lesions to biopsy. Carlens already pointed out the advantages of mediastinoscopy, not only as a staging procedure, but also as a diagnostic one for lung cancer and for other mediastinal diseases, such as lymphoma, lymph node metastasis from gastric and breast cancer, amyloidosis of the tracheal wall, and benign tracheal tumors. Reading Carlen's report more than half a century after publication gives the reader the impression of a very timely article and not of an outdated historical relic.

Indications and Contraindications

The European Society of Thoracic Surgeons (ESTS) has published guidelines on preoperative mediastinal staging in lung cancer that consider the computed tomography (CT) and the positron emission tomography (PET) or integrated PET-CT scans as leading imaging techniques in the staging process.[20] Any abnormality suggestive of N2 or N3 disease on CT has to undergo biopsy. Mediastinoscopy is the procedure of choice, but EBUS-FNA and EUS-FNA can provide cytologic confirmation that may be enough to start a multidisciplinary treatment protocol or to exclude resection. However, if these endoscopic procedures are negative, mediastinoscopy is still recommended, because the negative predictive value of EBUS-FNA and EUS-FNA is low. When there is no mediastinal abnormality on CT and the tumor is a peripheral T1N0M0 squamous cell carcinoma, mediastinal exploration can be avoided. However, in T1N0M0 tumors of other histologic types or more advanced tumors, mediastinoscopy is recommended. If the leading imaging technique is PET or PET-CT, any abnormal uptake suggestive of mediastinal nodal disease should undergo biopsy by mediastinoscopy or by endoscopic techniques, but if the latter are negative, a confirmatory mediastinoscopy is indicated. When there is no abnormal mediastinal uptake, exploration with mediastinoscopy is still indicated when there are signs of N1 disease, in central tumors, in tumors with low standardized uptake value, and in tumors with mediastinal nodes larger than 1.6 cm in the shortest diameter. In a recent prospective validation, sensitivity, specificity, and positive and negative predictive values of the ESTS guidelines were 0.84, 1, 1, and 0.94, respectively.[21] The ESTS guidelines are in full agreement with the evidence-based recommendations of the American College of Chest Physicians, which also recommend pathologic confirmation of CT and PET abnormalities, and the confirmation with mediastinoscopy of negative results from endoscopic techniques.[22]

There are no clear guidelines as to when to indicate mediastinoscopy for staging of mesothelioma. The most recent guidelines of the European Society of Medical Oncology indicate that mediastinoscopy may be useful for clinical staging and that inclusion of N2 tumors for pleuropneumonectomy is controversial, implying that N2 disease should be ruled out before indicating such an extensive operation.[23] As in lung cancer, nodal disease in mesothelioma has a deleterious effect on prognosis, although the differences between N1 and N2 disease are not as clear as they are in lung cancer.[24] The guidelines of the European Respiratory Society and of the ESTS recommend mediastinoscopy to exclude direct mediastinal involvement (T4) and mediastinal nodal disease (N2 and N3) in those patients who are candidates for radical resection or multimodality treatment.[25]

Mediastinal nodal disease adversely impacts prognosis of resected lung metastases.[26,27] It may be found in an average of 22% (11%–33%) of patients considered for metastasectomy in those published series that looked at this specific problem.[28] Patients with preoperative evidence of mediastinal nodal disease should be excluded from resection, and mediastinoscopy is the best way to explore the mediastinum and confirm or rule out nodal disease.[28] Mediastinal nodal involvement is found in 10% of patients who undergo mediastinoscopy after staging CT, and who are otherwise candidates for pulmonary metastasectomy.[29]

Extrathoracic carcinomas seldom involve mediastinal lymph nodes. In this circumstance, mediastinoscopy can be indicated to confirm diagnosis and stage the tumor spread, and also to assess resectability in selected cases.[30]

There are very few contraindications. Severe neck rigidity may prevent the right insertion of the mediastinoscope, but this is a rare circumstance that the authors have encountered only once in more than 2000 mediastinoscopies. Large goiters are an anatomic difficulty to the insertion of the instrument, and other alternative procedures should be used. This also is a rare circumstance. The normal thyroid gland and small goiters can be pushed cranially to allow the insertion of the mediastinoscope. As in all surgical procedures,

abnormal coagulation tests should be corrected before the intervention and are not real contraindications to the procedure. Other circumstances once considered contraindications are no longer contraindications. Mediastinoscopy can be performed safely after a previous mediastinoscopy and previous mediastinal operation through median sternotomy, in patients with superior vena cava syndrome, and in those with tracheostomy with total laryngectomy.[31,32]

Technique

Under general anesthesia and orotracheal intubation, the patient is positioned in the supine decubitus. A long sand or rubber cushion under the shoulders attains a slight hyperextension of the neck, exposing part of the intrathoracic trachea. The patient's head is allowed to rest on a circular rubber pillow to prevent lateral displacement of the head during the procedure (**Fig. 1**). The neck and the anterior chest wall from the mandible, cranially, to the xyphoid cartilage, caudally, and to the mid-clavicular lines, laterally, are prepared and draped as for median sternotomy. An additional drape covers the body of the sternum. This drape is easily removed if median sternotomy were necessary during the procedure. **Fig. 2** shows the basic instruments used during mediastinoscopy. **Fig. 3** shows the two more commonly used videomediastinoscopes.

For better comfort during the operation, the surgeon sits at the head of the operating table (**Fig. 4**). A 5-cm long collar incision is performed as close to the upper border of the manubrium as possible (**Fig. 5**A). The subcutaneous tissue and the platysma are incised, and dissection is performed deeply into the cervical midline. The paratracheal muscles and pretracheal fatty tissue

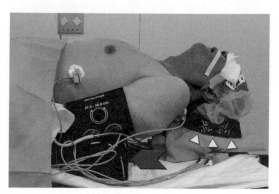

Fig. 1. Position of the patient for videomediastinoscopy. The cushion under the patient's shoulders raises the chest (*red arrow*). The neck is hyperextended and the head rests on a circular pillow (*yellow arrows*).

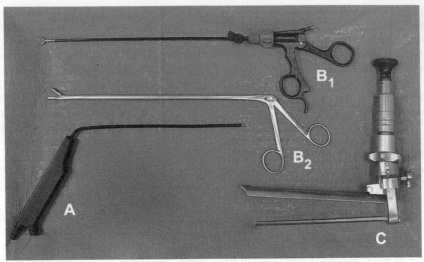

Fig. 2. Basic instrument set. (*A*) Dissection-coagulation-suction cannula. (*B₁*) Rotating biopsy forceps with connector pin for unipolar coagulation, size 5 mm. (*B₂*) Biopsy forceps with oval jaws, size 8 mm × 16 mm. (*C*) Two-bladed spreadable videomediastinoscope.

are separated laterally. At this point the anterior aspect of the trachea is seen (see **Fig. 5**B). The pretracheal fascia is held with forceps and incised with scissors. Then, the index finger is inserted into the incision and the pretracheal fascia is further torn caudally with finger dissection. Usually, after the distal phalange of the index finger is inserted into the incision, the pulsation of the innominate artery is felt. This is an anatomic landmark that can be compressed later with the mediastinoscope and the surgeon must be conscious of its location. In young or very flexible patients, the innominate artery becomes cervical after neck hyperextension and can be seen after incising

the platysma. It is important to bear this in mind to avoid injury during the initial neck dissection. The index finger is passed down into the mediastinum and behind the aortic arch, the pulsation of which can be clearly felt. The tracheal cartilages also can be felt. They split at the carina and in most patients this separation can be felt with finger palpation of the anterior wall of the trachea. Finger palpation provides the surgeon with information on tissue texture, size, and consistency of the peritracheal lymph nodes and on direct tumor involvement of the trachea or peritracheal tissue (**Fig. 6**).

Finger dissection has created an upper mediastinal space to insert the mediastinoscope, either under direct vision if a conventional scope is used, or watching the monitor if using a videomediastinoscope. Dissection of the peritracheal tissue is completed with the dissection-coagulation-suction device.

Mediastinoscopy for lung cancer staging should be thorough, but the thoroughness of the exploration may depend on its indication. If mediastinoscopy is indicated to confirm N3 disease, and confirmation is obtained by intraoperative frozen section, there is no need to continue the exploration unless the patient is in a protocol that requires more information. However, when there are no clear signs of mediastinal disease on CT or PET scans, mediastinoscopy should be systematic and complete. It is better to start by exploring and obtaining biopsy of the contralateral paratracheal nodes to rule out or confirm N3 disease, and then to proceed with the subcarinal nodes, and finally with the ipsilateral paratracheal nodes.

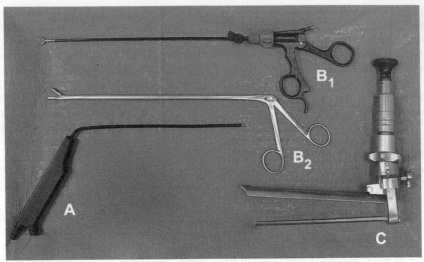

Fig. 3. Videomediastinoscopes. (*A*) Linder-Dahan videomediastinoscope. The dilating and parallel adjustable blades provide optimal three-dimensional space within the surgical field. (*B*) Lerut videomediastinoscope. The camera module is fully integrated in the handpiece so that the surgeon is able to work unhindered, even during the recording.

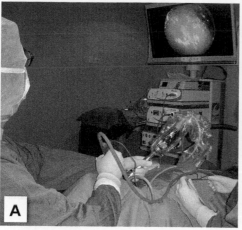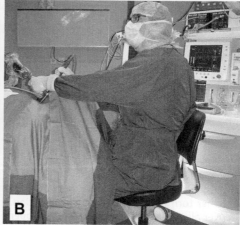

Fig. 4. Operating room view. (*A*) The monitor is located in front of the surgeon at the patient's feet and on the left. (*B*) The surgeon sits comfortably on a chair at the patient's head.

The ESTS guidelines determined that at least one node from the right and left inferior paratracheal and subcarinal nodes should undergo biopsy or be removed as the minimum requirement for an acceptable mediastinoscopy in routine clinical practice.[20] However, the right and left superior paratracheal nodes also are accessible to mediastinoscopy, but these rarely undergo biopsy because once the mediastinoscope is inserted into the mediastinum, they are excluded from the visual field by the mediastinoscope. Exploration and biopsy of these nodes are better done in the open fashion at the time of cervicotomy, and this maneuver should be done if there are radiographic or metabolic signs of nodal involvement at this level.

Mediastinoscopy allows the surgeon to explore the whole length of the trachea and both main bronchi. In light of the new lymph node map proposed by the International Association for the Study of Lung Cancer, some nodes that are anatomically located in the mediastinum are named hilar by international and multidisciplinary consensus. On the right side, those nodes caudal to the lower rim of the azygos vein should be labeled right hilar (#10R) nodes; on the left side, those caudal to the upper rim of the pulmonary artery should be labeled left hilar (#10L) nodes. Also, those located along the inferior aspects of both main bronchi and extending caudally to the end of the bronchus intermedius, on the right, and to the beginning of the left lower lobe bronchus, on the left, are all now subcarinal nodes (#7). Another important innovation of the new lymph node map is the shift of the mediastinal midline to the left paratracheal border. According to this, superior and inferior left paratracheal nodes are those intimately related to the left tracheal wall. To have proper access to them, the fibrous tissue layer that connects the pretracheal fascia

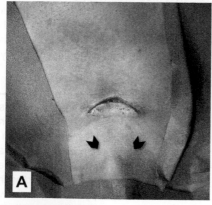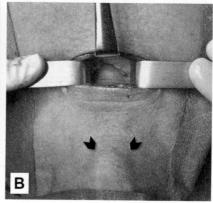

Fig. 5. (*A*) A 5-cm transverse incision is made above the superior margin of the sternum. (*B*) View of the trachea after the dissection and the lateral retraction of the pretracheal muscles (*arrows* show the thyroid cartilage).

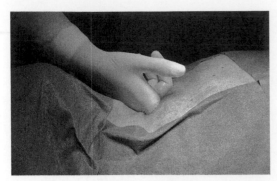

Fig. 6. Finger dissection and palpation. The index finger is inserted into the incision and the pretracheal fascia is further torn caudally with finger dissection. This maneuver allows the surgeon to create an upper mediastinal space to insert the mediastinoscope.

with the aorta has to be dissected. The nodes are found along the left tracheal wall in close relation with the left recurrent laryngeal nerve. All nodes anterior to this region, even if they are on the left of the mediastinal midline, are right superior or inferior paratracheal nodes (#2R or #4R nodes).[33] This new lymph node map has to be validated prospectively and does not imply any change in therapy derived from the change in nomenclature of the nodal stations.

Biopsy or removal of nodes may cause minor bleeding that can be controlled by gauze compression or by coagulation. Coagulation should be cautious on the left paratracheal margin to avoid injury to the left recurrent laryngeal nerve. Subcarinal nodes are vascularized by bronchial arteries and may bleed more than other mediastinal nodes. Clipping of the bronchial artery may be necessary to stop bleeding. The gauze used for hemostasis should be removed inside the mediastinoscope to avoid implantation of cancer cells in other parts of the mediastinum and in the cervical incision. Serious bleeding may occur if the vessels surrounding the operating field are injured: the innominate artery cranially; the superior vena cava and the azygos vein on the right; the ascending aorta and aortic arch anteriorly and on the left; and the right and left pulmonary arteries caudally, right on top of the subcarinal space. To avoid injury to these vessels, the surgeon should not lose eye contact with the anterior surface of the trachea and of the main bronchi, and should puncture any structure of dubious nature before obtaining from it a biopsy. This maneuver is especially useful if the conventional mediastinoscope is used, because its visual field is smaller than that of the videomediastinoscope. Care must be taken not to puncture through the tracheal wall to avoid perforation of the endotracheal tube.[34]

All biopsy sites should be checked for bleeding before closure. The peritracheal muscles are allowed to fall on their natural position and are not sutured to the midline. This makes remediastinoscopy easier if needed. The incision is closed in two layers with no drainage: platysma and subcutaneous tissue with continuous absorbable 2-0 sutures, and skin with intradermic 3-0 absorbable sutures (Movie 1).

In patients with left-sided lung cancer, if mediastinoscopy is negative, subaortic and para-aortic nodes must be explored.[20] This can be done by the traditional left parasternal mediastinotomy, by thoracoscopy, or by extended cervical mediastinoscopy.

Technical variants

Extended cervical mediastinoscopy From the mediastinoscopy incision, a passage is created by finger dissection over the aortic arch, between the innominate artery and the left carotid artery, either posteriorly or anteriorly to the left innominate vein. After the facia between both arteries is torn with the finger, the mediastinoscope is inserted obliquely and its tip reaches the subaortic space. Lymph nodes can be found among fatty tissue. The more anterior nodes are the para-aortic nodes, although the distinction between subaortic and para-aortic is not easy because the bony structures of the anterior chest wall limit the range of movement of the mediastinoscope (Movie 2).[35]

Mediastinoscopic biopsy of scalene lymph nodes If the mediastinoscope is passed behind the sternoclavicular insertion of the sternocleidomastoid muscles, the scalene lymph nodes can be reached and biopsied.[36]

Exploration of the right hilum Dissection of the right main bronchus allows biopsying the hilar nodes caudal to the azygos vein and posterior to the pulmonary artery.[37]

Inferior mediastinoscopy Inferior mediastinoscopy is performed by way of the subxiphoid approach. The indications are rare but it is worth having it in mind to biopsy mediastinal lesions that are out of the reach of cervical mediastinoscopy.[38,39]

Results

The virtues of mediastinoscopy in staging lung cancer are well established in the literature. In the past decade and a half, the introduction of the videomediastinoscope in clinical practice has prompted a series of comparative analyses to establish the relative value of conventional mediastinoscopy and videomediastinoscopy. **Table 1** shows results of recent series of conventional and videomediastinoscopies indicated for lung cancer staging.[40–45]

Table 1
Staging values of conventional mediastinoscopy and videomediastinoscopy

Author and Reference	Type of Mediastinoscopy	N	Sensitivity	Specificity	PPV	NPP	Diagnostic Accuracy
Rami-Porta & Mateu-Navarro,[40] 2002	CM	148	0.78	1	1	0.85	0.90
	VM	137	0.86	1	1	0.90	0.94
Venissac et al,[41] 2003	VM	240	0.91	1	1	NA	0.98
Lardinois et al,[42] 2003	VM with induction	24	0.81	1	1	NA	0.91
	VM without induction	195	0.87	1	1	NA	0.95
Leschber et al,[43] 2008	CM	52	NA	1	1	0.81	0.84
	VM	119	NA	1	1	0.83	0.88
Karfis et al,[44] 2008	VM	87	0.8	1	1	0.59	0.85
Anraku et al,[45] 2010	CM	505	0.92	1	1	0.95	0.97
	VM	140	0.95	1	1	0.98	0.98

Abbreviations: CM, conventional mediastinoscopy; N, number of patients; NA, not available; NPV, negative predictive value; PPV, positive predictive value; VM, videomediastinoscopy.

Rami-Porta and Mateu-Navarro[40] did not find any significant differences in the staging values of both procedures, although there was a tendency toward improved results with video-mediastinoscopy. Leschber and coworkers[43] observed lower rates of common complications in the videomediastinoscopy group, compared with the conventional mediastinoscopy group: 2.1% and 3% for recurrent laryngeal nerve palsy, respectively; and 0.9% and 2.3% for bleeding observed on postoperative chest radiograph, respectively. The mean number of biopsied or removed lymph nodes was greater in those patients who underwent videomediastinoscopy compared with those who underwent conventional mediastinoscopy: 8.1 and 6 lymph nodes, respectively. The same was true for those lymph nodes of the subcarinal station: 2.4 and 1.5, respectively. Negative predictive value and diagnostic accuracy for videomediastinoscopy tended to be better than for conventional mediastinoscopy: 0.83 and 0.81, and 0.88 and 0.84, respectively.[43] In the study by Anraku and colleagues,[45] no statistical differences were found in sensitivity, specificity, positive and negative predictive values, and accuracy of conventional mediastinoscopy and videomediastinoscopy, but the number of dissected lymph nodes (5 ± 2.8 and 7 ± 3.2, respectively; P<.001) and the number of nodal stations sampled (3.6 and 2.6, respectively; P<.001) were significantly higher for videomediastinoscopy. More recently, Cho and colleagues[46] compared the results of 222 conventional mediastinoscopies with those of 299 videomediastinoscopies and found a significantly lower complication rate (1.6% vs 3.6%; P = .03), a significantly higher number of dissected lymph nodes (8.53 ± 5.8 vs 7.13 ± 4.9; P = .004), and a significantly lower rate of recurrent laryngeal nerve palsy

(5.05 ± 4.5 vs 7.67 ± 6.5, respectively; P = .001) in videomediastinoscopies. However, there were no differences in the number of nodal stations explored. Although the videomediastinoscope is not strictly necessary to achieve a thorough, clinically acceptable mediastinoscopy, it has many advantages over the conventional one: larger and clearer images, the possibility to simultaneously share the procedure with trainees and all the personnel in the operative theater, the possibility to record the operation for future educational uses and discussion, and the possibility to improve its teaching without compromising the safety or completion of the procedure.[47]

Mediastinoscopy can be performed safely as an outpatient procedure. In a series of 50 mediastinoscopies for the diagnosis of hematologic malignancies, two (4%) patients were hospitalized because of pneumothorax and bleeding from a bronchial artery, requiring chest and wound drainages, respectively.[48] In a more recent series of 210 out-patient mediastinoscopies, only two patients (0.9%) required admission for treatment of pneumothorax and for late end of the operation, respectively.[49]

Table 2 summarizes the results of extended cervical mediastinoscopy for staging cancers of the left lung. The results are consistent in different institutions, and the negative predictive value generally is greater than 0.9.[35,50–53]

Complications

Intraoperative complications are rare and range from 0.6% to 3.7%.[54,55] Compression of the innominate artery is frequent, but can be easily controlled by fixing the pulse meter in one of the

Table 2
Staging values of published series of extended cervical mediastinoscopies

	Ginsberg et al[35]	López et al[50]	Freixinet et al[51]	Metin et al[52]	Obiols et al[53]
N	100	46	106	55	221
Sensitivity	0.69	0.83	0.81	0.69	0.67
Specificity	1	1	1	1	1
Accuracy	0.91	0.98	0.95	0.91	0.94
PPV	1	1	1	1	1
NPV	0.89	0.97	0.91	0.89	0.95

Abbreviations: N, number of patients; NPV, negative predictive value; PPV, positive predictive value.

right-hand fingers. After the pulse wave is absent, the surgeon has to reposition the mediastinoscope to relieve pressure on the artery. Bleeding from a big vessel is a rare but potentially fatal complication. It occurred in 14 (0.4%) out of 3391 patients who underwent the procedure, and the most common sites of bleeding were the azygos vein and the innominate and pulmonary arteries. In this series, packing followed by sternotomy was the most common procedure to control bleeding. There were no intraoperative deaths, but one patient died postoperatively.[56] Injury to the tracheobronchial tree may occur in 0.1% of patients (2 of 1743), but can usually be managed intraoperatively either by suturing or gluing the injury.[57] The left recurrent laryngeal nerve may be damaged by direct injury or by traction when the mediastinoscope goes under the aortic arch.[58] Chylomediastinum and chylothorax have been described after mediastinoscopy but are rare, at least those of clinical relevance.[59] Other complications include pneumothorax, wound infection, mediastinitis, esophageal perforation, and tumor implantation at the cervicotomy site.[60,61] Mortality ranges from 0% (no mortality in 4134 mediastinoscopies)[62] to 0.3% (1 in 324).[63]

REMEDIASTINOSCOPY
Historical Note

Palva[64] described the first remediastinoscopy in 1974. The case was not easy: fibrous scar tissue had developed between the innominate artery and the trachea and it was hard to develop a passage into the mediastinum. Based on this single case out of 330 mediastinoscopies, it was thought that remediastinoscopies should be contraindicated.[64] However, a year later, Palva and colleagues[65] published a report on six (0.5%) remediastinoscopies in their series of 1188 mediastinoscopies, and the fate of the exploration changed. The indications of these six remediastinoscopies were delayed therapy

in one, control of progressive disease diagnosed as nonmalignant at first mediastinoscopy in four, and recurrent tumor in one. The authors already described how useful it was to create a tunnel by digital palpation along the left (in two cases) or right (one case) side of the trachea to avoid the pretracheal adhesions, and to turn on top of the trachea when the mediastinoscope was already inserted into the mediastinum. No doubt this paper prompted other authors to perform remediastinoscopy and to extend its indications.

Indications and Contraindications

Since the publication by Palva and colleagues,[65] remediastinoscopy has been indicated in the following circumstances: inadequate first mediastinoscopy,[66–68] second primaries or recurrent lung cancers,[67–71] and staging of lung cancer after unrelated disease and other non–lung cancer diseases.[67] However, in the past decade, the most common indication has been the assessment of objective tumor response and downstaging of locally advanced lung cancer treated with induction therapy.[67,68,71–78] A third mediastinoscopy is a rare occurrence, but it has been proved to be feasible.[68,79] The ESTS guidelines on preoperative staging recommend remediastinoscopy to assess objective tumor response after induction therapy, unless an endoscopic procedure with FNA has yielded a positive result.[20]

Evident progressive local or distant disease during induction therapy is not common, but it should be diagnosed by the least invasive method. At remediastinoscopy, if firm adhesions are found in front of the trachea and a passage cannot be developed on either side of the trachea, it is better to terminate the operation and proceed with resection if there are no clear signs of persistent nodal disease, or rely on another staging method if there are such signs. This is a rare circumstance that the authors have encountered only once in more than 100 remediastinoscopies for several indications.

Technique

In principle, the technique does not differ much from mediastinoscopy. The main objective of remediastinoscopy is to take new biopsies of those nodes that had been positive at mediastinoscopy. Remediastinoscopy should be performed by the same surgeon who performed mediastinoscopy. If this is not possible, surgery and pathology records should be read for information regarding the extent of the original exploration and the location of the positive nodes. CT and PET scans should be readily available to identify the possible location of persistent nodal disease.

After resection of the previous surgical scar, dissection is performed deeply through the midline. Because the paratracheal muscles were not sutured to the midline, this poses no difficulty. However, the pretracheal fascia is invariably thickened and cannot be separated from the trachea as easily as at mediastinoscopy. There always are peritracheal adhesions, the consistency of which

varies from patient to patient. These are best managed by finger dissection. Contrary to what one might think, these adhesions rarely bleed. With finger dissection, as much peritracheal space as possible is created to allow the insertion of the mediastinoscope. The remaining adhesions are freed with instrumental dissection, using the dissection-coagulation-suction device or bipolar scissors. In the typical case, more adhesions are found along the right paratracheal margin. This is an area that harbors more nodes than its left counterpart, and more dissection and manipulation is performed at mediastinoscopy. It is recommended, as Palva and colleagues[65] described, to insert the mediastinoscope along the left paratracheal margin and change its position toward the anterior surface of the trachea and the right paratracheal margin after the scope is in the mediastinum (**Fig. 7**). The nodal station with positive nodes at mediastinoscopy should be explored first. If residual nodes are found, these should be rebiopsied and sent for frozen section. If tumor persists, the operation can be terminated, unless a specific protocol requires additional information of the extent of residual nodal involvement after

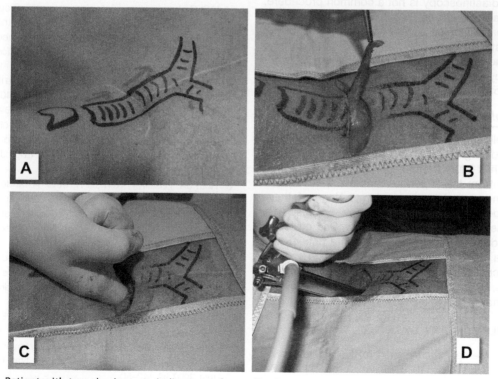

Fig. 7. Patient with two classic contraindications of remediastinoscopy: a previous mediastinoscopy and previous mediastinal surgery (median sternotomy for resection of bilateral lung cancer). Remediastinoscopy was indicated to rule out mediastinal nodal disease when a left upper lobe lesion was suspected of recurrent tumor. (*A*) Operative field showing previous mediastinoscopy and median sternotomy incisions. (*B*) Resection of previous mediastinoscopy incision scar. (*C*) Digital dissection along the left paratracheal margin. (*D*) Insertion of videomediastinoscope along the left paratracheal margin.

Table 3
Restaging values of remediastinoscopy

	Mateu-Navarro et al[72]	Van Schil et al[73]	Stamatis et al[74]	De Leyn et al[75]	De Waele et al[76]	Marra et al[77]	Call et al[68]
N	24	27	165	30	104	104	83
Sensitivity	0.7	0.73	0.74	0.29	0.71	0.61	0.74
Specificity	1	1	1	1	1	1	1
Accuracy	0.8	0.85	0.92	0.60	0.84	0.88	0.87
PPV	1	1	1	1	1	1	1
NPV	0.58	0.75	0.86	0.52	0.73	0.85	0.79

Abbreviations: N, number of patients; NPV, negative predictive value; PPV, positive predictive value.

induction therapy. When persistent nodal disease is not evident or is not proved by frozen section, remediastinoscopy should be as thorough as the anatomy permits. At the end of the operation, all biopsy sites should be checked for hemostasis and the incision is closed in two layers with no drainage.

Results

Remediastinoscopy is not a common procedure, but **Table 3** shows that it can be performed in different countries and by different surgeons with consistent results. Its results do not seem to depend on the type of induction therapy (chemotherapy or chemoradiation) or on the thoroughness of the initial mediastinoscopy.[68]

Complications

Complications include wound infection, unintended lung biopsy with no further consequences, bronchial injury treated with sealant, and hemorrhage from the superior vena cava that required packing and right thoracotomy. None of these are specific of remediastinoscopy, because they can also occur at mediastinoscopy. One intraoperative death has been described in a patient who was a poor candidate for an induction therapy protocol. Considering the four largest published series, this intraoperative death represents a mortality rate of 0.2%.[68,74,75,78]

SUPPLEMENTARY DATA

Supplementary data related to this article can be found online at doi:10.1016/j.thorsurg.2011.12.003.

REFERENCES

1. Rusch VW, Crowley J, Giroux DJ, et al. The IASLC lung cancer staging project: proposals for the revision of the N descriptors in the forthcoming seventh edition of the TNM classifications for lung cancer. J Thorac Oncol 2007;2:603–12.
2. Shepherd FA, Crowley J, Van Houtte P, et al. The International Association for the Study of Lung Cancer lung cancer staging project: proposals regarding the clinical staging of small cell lung cancer in the forthcoming (seventh) edition of the tumor, node, metastasis classification for lung cancer. J Thorac Oncol 2007;2:1067–77.
3. Vallières E, Shepherd FA, Crowley J, et al. The IASLC lung cancer staging project. Proposals regarding the relevance of the TNM in the pathologic staging of small cell lung cancer in the forthcoming (seventh) edition of the TNM classification for lung cancer. J Thorac Oncol 2009;4:1049–59.
4. Mountain CF. The biological operability of stage III non-small cell lung cancer. Ann Thorac Surg 1985;40:60–4.
5. Rosell R, Gomez-Codina J, Camps C, et al. A randomized trial comparing preoperative chemotherapy plus surgery with surgery alone in patients with non-small cell lung cancer. N Engl J Med 1994;330:153–8.
6. Roth JA, Fosella F, Komaki R, et al. A randomized trial comparing perioperative chemotherapy and surgery with surgery alone in resectable stage IIIA non-small cell lung cancer. J Natl Cancer Inst 1994;86:673–80.
7. Song WA, Zhou NK, Wang W, et al. Survival benefit of neoadjuvant chemotherapy in non-small cell lung cancer. An updated meta-analysis of 13 randomized control trials. J Thorac Oncol 2010;5:510–6.
8. Van Meerbeeck JP, Kramer GW, van Schil PE, et al. Randomized controlled trial of resection versus radiotherapy after induction chemotherapy in stage IIIA-N2 non-small-cell lung cancer. J Natl Cancer Inst 2007;99:442–50.
9. Albain KS, Swan RS, Rusch VW, et al. Radiotherapy plus chemotherapy with or without surgical resection for stage III non-small cell lung cancer: a phase III randomised controlled trial. Lancet 2009;374:379–86.

10. Van Schil P. The restaging issue. Lung Cancer 2003; 42(Suppl 1):s39–45.

11. Ernst A, Feller-Kopman D, Herth FJ. Endobronchial ultrasound in the diagnosis and staging of lung cancer and other thoracic malignancies. Semin Thorac Cardiovasc Surg 2007;19:201–5.

12. Talebian M, van Bartheld MB, Braun J, et al. EUS-FNA in the preoperative staging of non-small cell lung cancer. Lung Cancer 2010;69:60–5.

13. Hürtgen M, Friedel G, Toomes H, et al. Radical video-assisted mediastinoscopic lymphadenectomy (VAMLA): technique and first results. Eur J Cardiothorac Surg 2002;21:348–51.

14. Leschber G, Holinka G, Linder A. Video-assisted mediastinoscopic lymphadenectomy (VAMLA): a method for systematic mediastinal lymph node dissection. Eur J Cardiothorac Surg 2003;24:192–5.

15. Zielinski M. Transcervical extended mediastinal lymphadenectomy: results of staging in two hundred fifty-six patients with non-small cell lung cancer. J Thorac Oncol 2007;2:370–2.

16. Carlens E. Mediastinoscopy: a method for inspection and tissue biopsy in the superior mediastinum. Dis Chest 1959;4:343–52.

17. Daniels AC. A method of biopsy useful in diagnosing certain intrathoracic diseases. Dis Chest 1949;16:360–7.

18. Harken DE, Black H, Clauss R, et al. A simple cervicomediastinal exploration for tissue diagnosis of intrathoracic disease. N Engl J Med 1954;251:1041–4.

19. Radner S. Suprasternal node biopsy in lympha-spreading intrathoracic disease. Acta Med Scand 1955;152:413–5.

20. De Leyn P, Lardinois D, Van Schil PE, et al. ESTS guidelines for preoperative lymph node staging for non-small cell lung cancer. Eur J Cardiothorac Surg 2007;32:1–8.

21. Gunluoglu MZ, Melek H, Medetoglu B, et al. The validity of preoperative lymph node staging guidelines of European Society of Thoracic Surgeons in non-small-cell lung cancer patients. Eur J Cardiothorac Surg 2011;40:287–90.

22. Detterbeck FC, Jantz MA, Wallace M, et al. Invasive mediastinal staging of lung cancer. ACCP evidence-based clinical practice guidelines (2nd edition). Chest 2007;132:202S–20S.

23. Stahel RA, Weder W, Lievens Y, et al. Malignant pleural mesothelioma: ESMO clinical practice guidelines for diagnosis, treatment and follow-up. Ann Oncol 2010;21(Suppl 5):v126–8.

24. Rusch V, Giroux D, Kennedy K, et al. Initial analysis of IASLC mesothelioma database. J Thorac Oncol 2011;6(Suppl):s406.

25. Scherpereel A, Astoul P, Baas P, et al. Guidelines of the European Respiratory Society and the European Society of Thoracic Surgeons for the management of malignant pleural mesothelioma. Eur Respir J 2010; 35:479–95.

26. Pfannschmidt J, Klode J, Muley T, et al. Nodal involvement at the time of pulmonary metastasectomy: experience in 245 patients. Ann Thorac Surg 2006;81:448–54.

27. Welter S, Jacobs J, Krbek T, et al. Prognostic impact of lymph node involvement in pulmonary metastasis from colorectal cancer. Eur J Cardiothorac Surg 2007;31:167–72.

28. García-Yuste M, Cassivi S, Paleru C. Thoracic lymphatic involvement in patients having pulmonary metastasectomy. Incidence and the effect on prognosis. J Thorac Oncol 2010;5:s166–9.

29. Menon A, Milton R, Thorpe JA, et al. The value of video-assisted mediastinoscopy in pulmonary metastasectomy. Eur J Cardiothorac Surg 2007;32: 351–4.

30. Riquet M, Berna P, Brian E, et al. Intrathoracic lymph node metastases from extrathoracic carcinoma: the place for surgery. Ann Thorac Surg 2009;88:200–5.

31. Dosios T, Theakos N, Chatziantoniou C. Cervical mediastinoscopy and anterior mediastinotomy in superior vena cava obstruction. Chest 2005;128:1551–6.

32. Yamada K, Kumar P, Goldstraw P. Cervical mediastinoscopy after total laryngectomy and radiotherapy: its feasibility. Eur J Cardiothorac Surg 2002;21:71–3.

33. Rusch VW, Asamura H, Watanabe H, et al. The IASLC lung cancer staging project. A proposal for a new international lymph node map in the forthcoming seventh edition of the TNM classification for lung cancer. J Thorac Oncol 2009;4:568–77.

34. Mavridou P, Papadopoulou M, Igropoulou O, et al. Unexpected endotracheal tub cuff perforation during video mediastinoscopy. J Cardiothorac Vasc Anesth 2007;21:723.

35. Ginsberg RJ, Rice TW, Goldberg M, et al. Extended cervical mediastinoscopy. A single staging procedure for bronchogenic carcinoma of the left upper lobe. J Thorac Cardiovasc Surg 1987;94:673–8.

36. Lee JD, Ginsberg RJ. Lung cancer staging: the value if ipsilateral scalene lymph node biopsy performed at mediastinoscopy. Ann Thorac Surg 1996;62:338–41.

37. Chen C, Zhou YM. Extended mediastinoscopic examination at the right hilum. Ann Thorac Surg 2008;86:1704–6.

38. Arom KV, Franz JL, Grover FL, et al. Subxiphoid anterior mediastinal exploration. Ann Thorac Surg 1977;24: 289–90.

39. Hutter J, Junger W, Miller K, et al. Subxiphoidal videomediastinoscopy for diagnostic access to the anterior mediastinum. Ann Thorac Surg 1998;66: 1427–8.

40. Rami-Porta R, Mateu-Navarro M. Videomediastinoscopy. J Bronchol 2002;9:138–44.

41. Venissac N, Alifano M, Mouroux J. Video-assisted mediastinoscopy: experience from 240 consecutive cases. Ann Thorac Surg 2003;76:208–12.

42. Lardinois D, Schallberger A, Betticher D, et al. Post-induction video-mediastinoscopy is as accurate and safe as video-mediastinoscopy in patients without pretreatment for potentially operable non-small cell lung cancer. Ann Thorac Surg 2003;75:1102–6.

43. Leschber G, Sperling D, Klemm W, et al. Does video-mediastinoscopy improve the results of conventional mediastinoscopy? Eur J Cardiothorac Surg 2008;33:289–93.

44. Karfis EA, Roustanis E, Beis J, et al. Video-assisted cervical mediastinoscopy: our seven-year experience. Interact Cardiovasc Thorac Surg 2008;7:1015–8.

45. Anraku M, Miyata R, Compeau C, et al. Video-assisted mediastinoscopy compared with conventional mediastinoscopy: are we doing better? Ann Thorac Surg 2010;89:1577–81.

46. Cho JH, Kim J, Kim K, et al. A comparative analysis of video-assisted mediastinoscopy and conventional mediastinoscopy. Ann Thorac Surg 2011;92:1007–11.

47. Martin-Ucar AE, Chetty GK, Vaughan R, et al. A prospective audit evaluating the role of video-assisted cervical mediastinoscopy (VAM) as a training tool. Eur J Cardiothorac Surg 2004;26:393–5.

48. Venuta F, Rendina EA, Pescarmona EO, et al. Ambulatory mediastinal biopsy for hematologic malignancies. Eur J Cardiothorac Surg 1997;11:218–21.

49. Molins L, Fibla JJ, Pérez J, et al. Outpatient thoracic surgical programme in 300 patients: clinical results and economic impact. Eur J Cardiothorac Surg 2006;29:271–5.

50. Lopez L, Varela A, Freixinet J, et al. Extended cervical mediastinoscopy: prospective study of fifty cases. Ann Thorac Surg 1994;57:555–7.

51. Freixinet Gilart J, García PG, de Castro FR, et al. Extended cervical mediastinoscopy in the staging of bronchogenic carcinoma. Ann Thorac Surg 2000;70:1641–3.

52. Metin M, Citak N, Sayar A, et al. The role of extended cervical mediastinoscopy in staging of non-small cell lung cancer of the left lung and a comparison with integrated positron emission tomography and computed tomography: does integrated positron emission tomography and computed tomography reduce the need for invasive procedures? J Thorac Oncol 2011;6:1713–9.

53. Obiols C, Call S, Rami-Porta R, et al. Extended cervical mediastinoscopy: mature results of a clinical protocol for staging bronchogenic carcinoma of the left lung. Eur J Cardiothorac Surg, in press.

54. Hammoud ZT, Anderson RC, Meyers BF, et al. The current role of mediastinoscopy in the evaluation of thoracic diseases. J Thorac Cardiovasc Surg 1999;118:894–9.

55. Kliems G, Savic B. Complications of mediastinoscopy. Endoscopy 1979;1:9–12.

56. Park BJ, Flores R, Downey RJ, et al. Management of major hemorrhage during mediastinoscopy. J Thorac Cardiovasc Surg 2003;126:726–31.

57. Saumench-Perramon R, Rami-Porta R, Call-Caja S, et al. Mediastinoscopic injuries to the right main bronchus and their mediastinoscopic repair. J Bronchol 2008;15:191–3.

58. Benouaich V, Marcheix B, Carfagna L, et al. Anatomical bases of left recurrent nerve lesions during mediastinoscopy. Surg Radiol Anat 2009;31:295–9.

59. Le Pimpec Barthes F, D'Attellis N, Assouad J, et al. Chylous leak after cervical mediastinoscopy. J Thorac Cardiovasc Surg 2003;126:1199–200.

60. Pereszlenyi A Jr, Niks M, Danko J, et al. Complications of video-mediastinoscopy: successful management in four cases. Bratisl Lek Listy 2003;104:201–4.

61. Pop D, Nadeemy AS, Venissac N, et al. Late mediastinal hematoma followed by incisional metastasis after video-assisted mediastinoscopy. J Thorac Oncol 2010;5:919–20.

62. Jepsen O. Mediastinoscopy. Copenhagen (Denmark): Munksgaard; 1966.

63. Urschel JD. Conservative management (packing) of hemorrhage complicating mediastinscopy. Ann Thorac Cardiovasc Surg 2000;6:9–12.

64. Palva T. Mediastinoscopy. Basel (Switzerland): S Karger; 1974.

65. Palva T, Palva A, Kärjä J. Remediastinoscopy. Arch Otolaryngol 1975;101:748–50.

66. Olsen PS, Stentoft P, Ellefsen B, et al. Remediastinoscopy in the assessment of resectability of lung cancer. Eur J Cardiothorac Surg 1997;11:661–3.

67. De Waele M, Hendriks J, Lauwers P, et al. Different indications for repeat mediastinoscopy: single institution experience of 79 cases. Minerva Chir 2009;64:415–8.

68. Call S, Rami-Porta R, Obiols C, et al. Repeat mediastinoscopy in all its indications: experience with 96 patients and 101 procedures. Eur J Cardiothorac Surg 2011;39:1022–7.

69. Lewis RJ, Sisler GE, Mackenzie JW. Repeat mediastinoscopy. Ann Thorac Surg 1984;37:147–9.

70. Meerschaut D, Vermassen F, Brutel de la Riviere A, et al. Repeat mediastinoscopy in the assessment of new and recurrent lung neoplasm. Ann Thorac Surg 1992;53:120–2.

71. Pauwels M, Van Schil P, De Backer W, et al. Repeat mediastinoscopy in the staging of lung cancer. Eur J Cardiothorac Surg 1998;14:271–3.

72. Mateu-Navarro M, Rami-Porta R, Bastus-Piulats R, et al. Remediastinoscopy after induction chemotherapy in non-small cell lung cancer. Ann Thorac Surg 2000;70:391–5.

73. Van Schil P, van der Schoot J, Poniewierski J, et al. Remediastinoscopy after neoadjuvant therapy for

non-small cell lung cancer. Lung Cancer 2002;37: 281–5.

74. Stamatis G, Fechner S, Hillejan L, et al. Repeat mediastinoscopy as a restaging procedure. Pneumologie 2005;59:862–6.

75. De Leyn P, Stroobants S, De Wever W, et al. Prospective comparative study of integrated positron emission tomography-computed tomography scan compared with remediastinoscopy in the assessment of residual mediastinal lymph node disease after induction chemotherapy for mediastinoscopy-proven stage IIIA-N2 non-small cell lung cancer: a Leuven Lung Cancer Group Study. J Clin Oncol 2006;24:3333–9.

76. De Waele M, Hendriks J, Lauwers P, et al. Nodal status at repeat mediastinoscopy determines survival in non-small cell lung cancer with mediastinal nodal involvement, treated by induction therapy. Eur J Cardiothorac Surg 2006;29:240–3.

77. Marra A, Hillejan L, Fechner S, et al. Remediastinoscopy in restaging of lung cancer after induction therapy. J Thorac Cardiovasc Surg 2008; 135:843–9.

78. De Waele M, Serra-Mitjans M, Hendriks J, et al. Accuracy and survival of repeat mediastinoscopy after induction therapy for non-small cell lung cancer in a combined series of 104 patients. Eur J Cardiothorac Surg 2008;33:824–32.

79. Schepens MA, Brutel de la Rivière A, Van den Bosch JM. Is a third mediastinoscopy really useful? Eur J Cardiothorac Surg 1995;9:612–4.

Ultrasound-Guided Transbronchial and Transesophageal Needle Biopsy in the Mediastinal Staging of Lung Cancer

Jarosław Kużdżał, MD, PhD, FETCS[a,*],
Artur Szlubowski, MD, PhD[b]

KEYWORDS

- Lung cancer • Mediastinum
- Endobronchial ultrasonography
- Endoscopic ultrasonography • Biopsy

The importance of mediastinal staging of lung cancer in clinical decision making is beyond any doubt. Recently, a rapid development of new techniques and strategies aimed at precisely establishing the stage of the disease, which in turn dictates the treatment option, has been witnessed. Widespread use of positron emission tomography/computed tomography (PET-CT) increased the demand for tissue diagnosis of lesions that were PET positive. There were, generally, 2 concepts of bioptic techniques: the maximally invasive and the minimally invasive techniques. The first concept comprises extensive surgical lymph node dissection, video-assisted mediastinal lymphadenectomy (VAMLA),[1] and transcervical extended mediastinal lymphadenectomy (TEMLA).[2] The second concept includes needle biopsy guided by endosonographic imaging, ie, endobronchial ultrasonography-guided needle aspiration (EBUS-NA) and endoscopic ultrasonography-guided needle aspiration (EUS-NA). As more data were published, TEMLA turned out to be associated with high mortality and complication rates that were unacceptable.[3] Simultaneously, technical progress led to the refinement of EBUS-NA and EUS-NA. For

these 2 reasons, these techniques are now becoming the primary methods of mediastinal lymph node biopsy in patients with lung cancer. This review is dedicated to endosonography-guided needle biopsy of mediastinal nodes and includes the technique, diagnostic yield, economic aspects, and future perspectives of real-time EBUS-NA and EUS-NA. The use of blind transbronchial NA and radial probe imaging are not discussed here; moreover, an assessment of the primary tumor and distant metastases is beyond the scope of this review.

EBUS
Equipment

There are several types of commercially available ultrasound videobronchoscopes, manufactured by Olympus, Pentax, and Fujinon. An ultrasound videobronchoscope has an outer diameter of 6.9 to 7.0 mm, a 2.0- to 2.2-mm working channel, and a 35° forward oblique-viewing optical system. Ultrasound processors are used for scanning at a frequency of 5 to 12 MHz, enabling a 20- to 100-mm depth tissue imaging. An electronic curved linear array ultrasonic transducer is

[a] Department of Thoracic Surgery, John Paul II Hospital, Jagiellonian University, 80 Pradnicka Street, 31-202 Cracow, Poland
[b] Endoscopy Unit, John Paul II Hospital, 80 Pradnicka Street, 31-202 Cracow, Poland
* Corresponding author.
E-mail address: j.kuzdzal@mp.pl

Thorac Surg Clin 22 (2012) 191–203
doi:10.1016/j.thorsurg.2011.12.006
1547-4127/12/$ – see front matter © 2012 Elsevier Inc. All rights reserved.

mounted at the distal end of the bronchoscope (**Fig. 1**) and may be covered by a water-inflatable balloon as an option for better visualization of nodes, but most bronchoscopists do not use it routinely. Image processing is performed by an endoscopic ultrasound center. For the biopsy, a cytologic 22- or 21-gauge needle with guide wire and marking facilitating its visualization on the ultrasound image is used. The currently available needles are 40 mm long and make it possible to puncture nodes located at a distance from the tracheal or bronchial wall (**Fig. 2**). Fine-NA is performed by passing the needle through the tracheal or bronchial wall and into the lymph nodes under real-time ultrasound control. Needle punctures are usually performed using the jabbing method. Integrated color- and power-Doppler mode can be used to identify mediastinal vessels immediately before needle puncture.

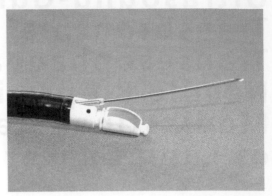

Fig. 2. A 40-mm long needle used for EBUS-NA.

Patient Preparation

Informed consent should be obtained from all patients, according to institutional regulations. Venous access should be secured. Patient monitoring includes electrocardiogram and pulse oximetry. Oxygen supplementation via nasal catheter is recommended.

Initially, EBUS was performed under general anesthesia with tracheal intubation. The present practice uses local anesthesia and conscious sedation using fentanyl (0.05–0.1 mg) and midazolam (1–5 mg). This approach makes it possible to perform EBUS in an outpatient setting, is safe, and reduces the use of hospital resources.

Technique

As the ultrasound bronchoscope is not designed for detailed assessment of the bronchial tree, the examination should be preceded by the standard

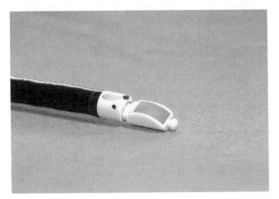

Fig. 1. Ultrasound bronchoscope equipped with a curved linear array ultrasonic transducer.

videobronchoscopy. Analysis of CT scans or PET-CT, if available, is done before the procedure to obtain as much information as possible regarding the anatomic relationships.

After the insertion of the EBUS endoscope into the trachea and visualizing the main carina, both the main bronchi are identified.

To enter the right main bronchus, the tip of the endoscope is levered and turned slightly to the right close to the lateral wall. After straightening the tip of the endoscope, having visualized but not entered the right upper lobe, the bronchoscope is moved into the intermediate bronchus, until the diameter of the bronchial tree prevents the endoscope from being advanced further. Usually this area is below the orifice of the middle- and lower-lobe bronchi, but the endoscope can sometimes be advanced further.

The described area just below the minor carina at the 2- to 4-o'clock position is adjacent to the right interlobar fissure and lymph nodes station 11R. A systematic endosonography staging should be started from this area. Withdrawal of the endoscope slightly and turning it to the 3-o'clock position just below the minor carina enables the endoscopist to visualize the remaining part of interlobar nodes (station 11R). The endoscope is withdrawn proximally to the entrance of the upper lobe of the right lung to the 2-o'clock position, which is adjacent to the right hilar lymph nodes (station 10R). After confirming the correct placement of the tip (ultrasonic transducer), the endoscopic image shows the minor carina, the bronchoscope is turned to the 9-o'clock position, and its tip is pressed against the bronchial wall of the right main bronchus just below the main carina; the ultrasonogram shows the subcarinal lymph nodes (station 7) (**Fig. 3**). After withdrawal of the bronchoscope proximally to the main carina and turning it to the 3-o'clock position, the right lower paratracheal lymph nodes (station 4R) are

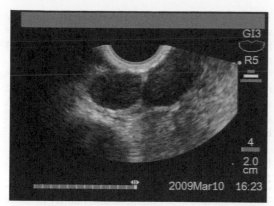

Fig. 3. EBUS image of metastatic subcarinal lymph nodes.

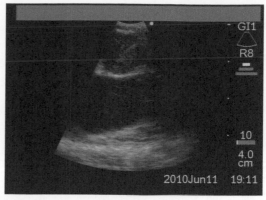

Fig. 5. EBUS-NA of the right upper paratracheal nodes adjacent to the superior vena cava.

visualized close to the superior vena cava and the azygos vein (**Fig. 4**). Above them, at the level of the middle trachea, right upper paratracheal lymph nodes (station 2R) are located (**Fig. 5**). By turning the endoscope to the 9-o'clock position on the contralateral side of the tracheal wall, left upper paratracheal lymph nodes (station 2L) can be scanned. A further rotation of the endoscope to the 6-o'clock position may visualize retrotracheal lymph nodes (station 3p); however, this is seldom possible.

Next, the endoscope is advanced to the left main bronchus, toward the carina between the upper and lower lobes of the left lung. As the tip of the endoscope is pressed against the bronchial wall at the 11-o'clock position, the area of the left hilar lymph nodes (station 10L) is visualized (**Fig. 6**). Rotation of the bronchoscope to the 2-o'clock position while approaching the proximal part of the left lower lobe bronchus shows the area of the left interlobar nodes (station 11L).

Then the bronchoscope is withdrawn slightly and its tip is pressed against the middle part of the lateral wall of the left main bronchus at the 9-o'clock position, to scan the area of the left lower paratracheal nodes (station 4L). The aortic arch can be followed posteriorly to the aortopulmonary (A-P) window; it is visualized proximally and the left pulmonary artery distally. Finally, the tip of the bronchoscope is turned to the 3-o'clock position and the subcarinal lymph nodes (station 7) are examined again from the left main bronchus.

The actual needle biopsy is performed with direct contact between the transducer and the wall of the trachea or bronchus. When a target lesion is visualized, a 22- or 21-gauge needle is introduced through the biopsy channel of the endoscope. A power- or color-Doppler examination may be performed to avoid an unintended puncture of a vessel, and the needle is advanced into the lesion under real-time ultrasound guidance (**Fig. 7**). Then suction is applied with a syringe, and the needle is moved back and forth inside the lesion.

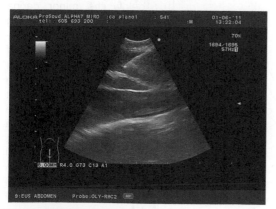

Fig. 4. EBUS-NA of the right lower paratracheal nodes located close to the superior vena cava just above the azygos vein.

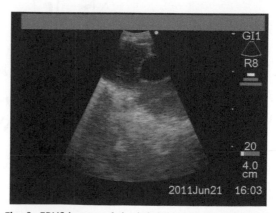

Fig. 6. EBUS image of the left hilar lymph nodes.

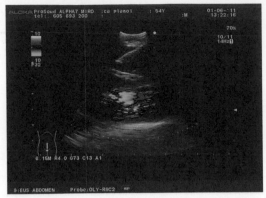

Fig. 7. EBUS-NA of the right lower paratracheal nodes. Color-Doppler imaging shows the superior vena cava.

EBUS-NA enables biopsy of stations 2R, 2L, 4R, 4L, and 7 (also N1 stations 10R, 10L, 11R, and 11L that are inaccessible for other invasive techniques, which is a unique advantage of EBUS-NA) (**Fig. 8, Table 1**).

The recommended number of needle passes depends on the presence or absence of a rapid on-site evaluation (ROSE) of the cytologic smears. The accuracy of EBUS-NA is related to the number of passes.[4] If ROSE is not available, we use 3 to 5 needle passes to obtain an optimal yield.

Handling of the Specimen

The aspirated specimen is placed on a glass slide and immediately fixed in 96% ethanol or sprayed with Cytofix. Standard hematoxylin-eosin (H&E) staining is used. The use of ROSE has the advantage of performing an additional biopsy if the initial specimen is insufficient to establish the diagnosis.

This technique has been shown to correlate very well with the final cytology.[5] The authors have found that the main cause for discrepancy was the scant cellularity of the specimen.

As an addition to the standard staining, immunohistochemical assays may be used.[6] Cytologic aspirates obtained using EBUS-NA or EUS-NA allow genetic evaluation, including K-ras,[7–10] EGFR,[7–12] and ALK.[13]

EUS
Equipment

The ultrasound videogastroscope has an external diameter of 12.3 to 14.6 mm, a working channel of 3.0 to 3.7 mm, and a 55° oblique anterior optical system. The electronic curved linear array ultrasonic transducer is mounted at the distal end (**Fig. 9**). Ultrasound processors are used for scanning at a frequency of 5 to 12 MHz, enabling 20- to 100-mm depth tissue imaging. For the biopsy, a cytologic, 80-mm long, 21/22-gauge needle or a histologic 19-gauge needle with guide wire and marking facilitating its visualization on the ultrasonogram may be used. Its length allows for a biopsy of structures located far away from the tracheal or bronchial wall (**Fig. 10**). Fine-NA is performed by passing the needle through the esophageal wall and into the lymph nodes under real-time ultrasound control. Integrated color- and power-Doppler mode can be used to identify mediastinal vessels immediately before needle puncture.

Patient Preparation

Patients' preparation and medication follows the same principles as described previously for EBUS-NA.

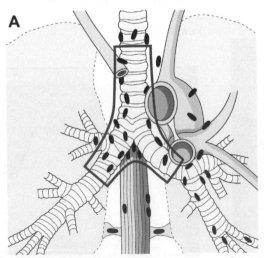
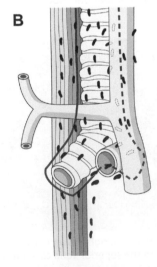

Fig. 8. The reach of EBUS-NA. (*A*) Anterior view; (*B*) lateral view.

Table 1
Accessibility of nodal stations using endosonography imaging and biopsy

Nodal Station	EBUS-NA	EUS-NA	CUS-NA
1	N	N	N
2	Y	Y	Y
3a	N	N	N
3p	Y/N	Y	Y
4	Y	Y	Y
5	N	Y[a]	Y[a]
6	N	N[b]	N[b]
7	Y[c]	Y[d]	Y
8	N	Y	Y
9	N	Y	Y
10	Y	N	Y
11	Y	N	Y

Abbreviations: Y, yes; N, no.
[a] Visualization of the whole station, biopsy of the lower part only.
[b] Visualization only.
[c] Better for the anterior part of station 7.
[d] Better for the posterior part of station 7.

Technique

The ultrasound videogastroscope is inserted through the mouth into the esophagus and advanced under visual control to the stomach. Starting from the gastric fundus, the intraluminal scanning guides the further procedure. At the cardia region, the transducer is turned until the abdominal aorta is clearly visualized in its longitudinal diameter. To visualize the left adrenal gland, the tip of the gastroscope is slid down the aorta up to the celiac trunk, which is the first vessel extending from the abdominal aorta. At this point, the endoscope is turned clockwise (this movement

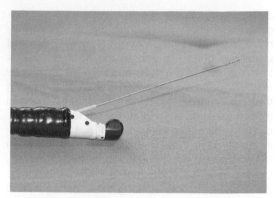

Fig. 10. An 80-mm long needle used for EBUS-NA enables biopsy of targets remote from the esophageal wall.

turns the transducer to the left) to visualize the left kidney, the spleen, and the left adrenal gland. After visualizing the left adrenal gland, the transducer is brought back to its standard position at the cardia. In front of it the left lobe of the liver is clearly visualized, and to the right the hepatic veins can be followed as they approach the inferior vena cava. Then the scanning proceeds by withdrawing the transducer to the distal esophagus; the EUS gastroscope is turned round (360°) from the descending aorta and back to the aorta again, visualizing retroperitoneal and para-aortic lymph nodes. If the gastroscope is turned slightly more to the left, a diaphragm is clearly seen on the left and the right atrium on the right, and left pulmonary ligament lymph nodes (station 9) may be examined. During withdrawal of the EUS scope from the distal to the middle part of the esophagus, paraesophageal lymph nodes (station 8) are seen posteriorly (**Fig. 11**), then the heart is visualized anteriorly with the left ventricle coming first into focus, then the atrioventricular valves and left

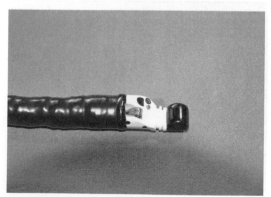

Fig. 9. Ultrasound gastroscope equipped with a curved linear array ultrasonic transducer.

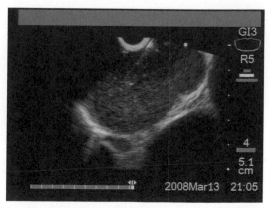

Fig. 11. EUS image of the paraesophageal lymph nodes.

atrium with pulmonary vein close to the esophageal wall; while withdrawing the scope slightly more, subcarinal lymph nodes (station 7) are well visualized (**Fig. 12**), and to the right reflections from the trachea are seen, and the right pulmonary artery in a transverse section is seen. Withdrawing the scope more and looking anterior at the tracheal reflections at its lower part, the left lower paratracheal lymph nodes (station 4L) (**Fig. 13**) and deeper aortic-pulmonary window (station 5) between the pulmonary artery and aorta are well visualized. On the left, the entire descending intrathoracic aorta can be followed along the esophagus, and para-aortic lymph nodes (station 6) may be visualized through the aortic arch. Behind the aorta, reflections from the thoracic spine are well visualized. As the gastroscope is withdrawn further, the subclavian artery and upper left paratracheal lymph nodes (station 2L) are visualized on the left side (**Fig. 14**), and just behind them the left the internal jugular vein is often seen. At the level of the upper part of the esophagus, both lobes of the thyroid gland can be seen.

The technique of the needle biopsy is similar to that described previously for EBUS-NA. However, the reach of EUS is different: it is possible to puncture the stations 2R and 2L, 3p, 4R, and 4L; the lower part of station 5; stations 7 (particularly its posterior part), 8, and 9 (**Fig. 15**, see **Table 1**).

COMBINED ULTRASONOGRAPHY

The main disadvantage of EBUS-NA and EUS-NA is the limited reach of each of these techniques. However, as shown in **Table 1** and **Fig. 16**, the reach of them is highly complementary. In 2005, Vilmann and colleagues[14] published the original series of 33 patients staged using combined EBUS-NA and EUS-NA.

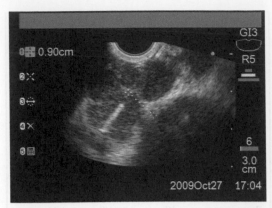

Fig. 13. EUS performed using the ultrasound bronchoscope showing the needle biopsy of the left lower paratracheal lymph nodes.

Equipment, preparation of the patient, and handling of the specimen are the same as described earlier. The technique of combined ultrasonography (CUS) and needle biopsy was initially a sum of both methods as described earlier. Because bronchoscopy has been the domain of pulmonologists and thoracic surgeons whereas endoscopy of the digestive tract has been the area of expertise of gastroenterologists and general surgeons, these 2 examinations were generally performed separately. However, thoracic surgeons and dedicated endoscopists, experienced in both bronchoscopy and esophagoscopy, perform both endoscopies as one procedure, usually with local anesthesia and conscious sedation. This strategy is better tolerated by patients, shortens the time needed to establish the final stage, and reduces the cost.

The next important step was the introduction of the single-scope CUS.[15,16] In this variation, EBUS

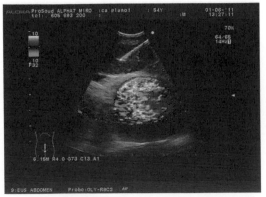

Fig. 12. EUS-NA of the subcarinal lymph nodes. Color-Doppler imaging shows the pulmonary artery.

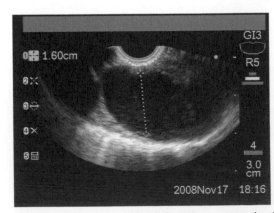

Fig. 14. EUS image of the left upper paratracheal lymph nodes.

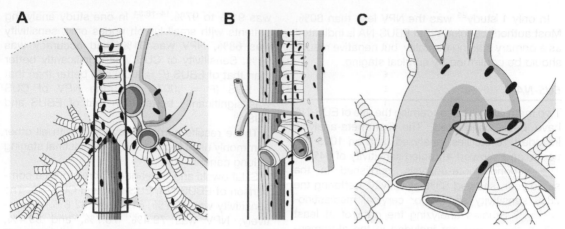

Fig. 15. The reach of EUS-NA. (*A*) Anterior view; (*B*) lateral view; (*C*) region of A-P window.

and EUS are performed using the same ultrasound bronchoscope. Although it does not allow for imaging and biopsy of the left adrenal gland or liver metastases, it is fully sufficient for mediastinal staging. Reduced length of time of the procedure and lower hospital costs are the advantages of this approach.[17]

DIAGNOSTIC YIELD
EBUS-NA

There have been 3 meta-analyses of studies on the diagnostic yield of EBUS-NA published to date. The first meta-analysis included 8 studies and data on 918 patients.[18] The sensitivity of EBUS-NA was 90%. The second meta-analysis included 10 studies and analyzed data on 782 patients.[19] The pooled sensitivity of EBUS-NA was 88%.

The investigators stressed the poor quality of the studies, and concluded that more data were needed regarding comparison of EBUS-NA with mediastinoscopy.

The last meta-analysis included 11 studies and 1299 patients, and showed a 93% sensitivity of EBUS-NA. All these results compare favorably with the sensitivity of standard cervical mediastinoscopy, which was 78% in a recent meta-analysis of data on 6505 patients.[18]

Several other studies, not included in the aforementioned meta-analyses, presented results of EBUS-NA in mediastinal staging of lung cancer. According to those including at least 100 patients, the sensitivity of EBUS-NA was 88.1% to 95.08%,[4,20–26] the negative predictive value (NPV) was 60% to 96.7%,[4,20,21,23–27] and the overall accuracy was 91.7% to 97.02%.[4,21,23–25]

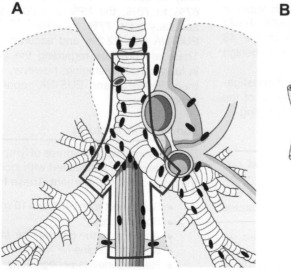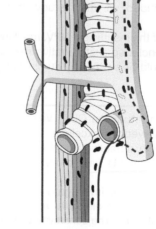

Fig. 16. The reach of CUS-NA. (*A*) Anterior view; (*B*) lateral view.

In only 1 study[25] was the NPV less than 80%. Most authors conclude that EBUS-NA is indicated as a primary staging modality, but negative results should be confirmed by surgical staging.

EUS-NA

Two meta-analyses concerning the use of EUS-NA have been conducted. The first meta-analysis included 16 studies, analyzed data on 1003 patients, and showed a pooled sensitivity of 84%.[18] The second meta-analysis, published in the same year, showed 83% sensitivity, bettering the 78% sensitivity shown for cervical mediastinoscopy.[18] Studies analyzing the data of at least 100 patients and not included in the aforementioned meta-analyses provide additional information. According to these studies the sensitivity of EUS-NA was 74% to 92%,[28–30] the NPV was 73%,[29] and accuracy was 83% to 93%.[29–31]

Witte and colleagues[32] analyzed the impact of such variables as size of the nodes, side of the primary tumor, and nodal station on the sensitivity of EUS-NA. These investigators found that the sensitivity was 91.7% for bulky nodes, 78.1% for nodes larger than 1 cm, and 43.8% for nodes normal on CT scans. The sensitivity was worse for right-sided tumors (50%) than for the left-sided tumors (96.6%). Also, nodal stations 7, 5/6, 4R, and 4L were associated with different sensitivity of EUS-NA, being 80.6%, 78.9%, 23.8%, and 25%, respectively.

Storch and colleagues[33] used large-bore needles for core-biopsy on lymph nodes in addition to EUS-NA. The overall accuracy of EUS-NA, large-bore needle biopsy, and the combination of both was 79%, 79%, and 98%, respectively. The investigators concluded that a combination of cytologic and histologic needle biopsy is superior to EBUS-NA alone. However, the results should be interpreted with caution, as 19 of the 48 patients included in their study had benign disease.

Because of the insufficient NPV, most investigators have concluded that negative results of the EUS-NA should be verified by surgical staging.

CUS-NA

In the original study on CUS, Vilmann and colleagues[14] showed an excellent diagnostic yield: the accuracy in detecting nodal metastases was 100% in 33 patients with proven or suspected lung cancer.

After that, several investigators published results of large studies aimed to assess the diagnostic yield of CUS. The sensitivity was 91.1% to 93%, the NPV was 91% to 97%, and accuracy was 91% to 97%.[14–16,34] In one study analyzing patients with small lymph nodes only, sensitivity was 68%, NPV was 91%, and accuracy was 91%. Sensitivity of CUS was significantly better than that of EBUS (P = .004) and better than that of EUS (P = .007). Also, the NPV of CUS was significantly better than that of EBUS and EUS.[35]

These results compare favorably with all other commonly used techniques of mediastinal staging of lung cancer.

Szlubowski and colleagues[36] presented a comparison of EBUS-NA, EUS-NA, and CUS-NA. The sensitivity was 62.7%, 61%, and 82.8%, respectively; NPV was 79.4%, 78.7%, and 89.4%, respectively; and the accuracy was 84.1%, 83.4% and 91.7%, respectively. Although the sensitivity of the EBUS-NA and EUS-NA did not differ significantly (P = .849), there were significant differences between CUS-NA and both EBUS-NA (P = .016) and EUS-NA (P = .010). Similarly, there was no significant difference between the NPV of EBUS-NA and EUS-NA (P = .089), but the NPV of CUS-NA was significantly better than that of EBUS-NA (P = .049) and EUS-NA (P = .042).

SPECIAL CONSIDERATIONS
Restaging

Restaging after induction therapy is a difficult and controversial issue. The sensitivity of imaging studies is lower than primary staging of lung cancer, and surgical staging is technically more complex and is associated with a higher risk of complications. This is particularly true if the primary staging was also surgical, because of the scarring on the mediastinum. The sensitivity of EBUS-NA in lung cancer restaging was 67% to 76%, the NPV was 20% to 78%, and accuracy was 77% to 80%.[37,38] The NPV of EUS-NA was 92.3% and accuracy was 91.6%. There are no data regarding the value of CUS in lung cancer restaging; however, results better than EBUS-NA and EUS-NA separately can be expected.

Sonographic Features

Several sonographic features of lymph nodes have been described, associated with increased risk of their malignant involvement. These features are:

- Size (short axis >8.5 or >10 mm)
- Round shape
- Absence of the central hilar structure
- Distinct margins
- Heterogeneous echogenicity
- Coagulation necrosis sign.

In a large study, including analysis of sonographic features of 1061 lymph nodes, Fujiwara and colleagues[39] found that a short axis greater than 10 mm, round shape, and a distinct margin at the absence of the central hilar structure were independent prognostic factors of metastatic lymph node involvement. Gill and colleagues[40] also found the first 3 of these features to be independent prognosticators; however, they used a cutoff of 8.5 mm for the size of the node. In their series, 63% of nodes with all these 3 features were metastatic, but if none of them was present, only 4% contained metastatic deposits. Sawhney and colleagues[41] analyzed a group of 67 patients and found that absence of the central hilar structure (termed by the investigators "central intranodal vessel") had 75% sensitivity, 97% specificity, and 89% accuracy in predicting nodal metastases. The diagnostic value of this feature was superior to the shape, margin, and echogenicity.

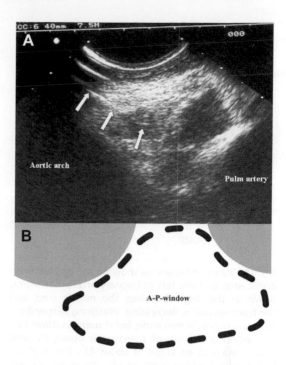

Fig. 17. (A) EUS image showing biopsy of nodes located between trachea and the plane of aortic arch/pulmonary artery, termed "nodes in the aorto-pulmonary window." Arrows indicate needle and needle tip in one of the nodes. (B) Extension drawing showing the true position of AP-window nodes, located far away from the region of biopsy performed.

The Question of the A-P Window Nodes

There has been a lot of misunderstanding regarding the accessibility of the A-P window nodes (station 5) using EBUS-NA and EUS-NA. During the last decade, several investigators described the transbronchial or transesophageal biopsy of these nodes. However, some of them did in fact puncture the left lower paratracheal (station 4L) nodes, misinterpreted as the A-P window. In some reports, biopsy of what was termed the A-P window was depicted (**Fig. 17A**). It should be remembered that the space between the tracheal and esophageal wall, aorta, and the left pulmonary artery is the location of station 4L, whereas the station 5 nodes are located in front of the plane of the aorta and pulmonary artery (see **Fig. 17B**).

According to data in the literature, the mean diameter of the aortic arch is 24 mm and that of the left pulmonary artery is 20 mm. The width of the gap between these vessels is 6 to 10 mm. However, the tracheal or esophageal wall is never punctured at a right angle; the needle always passes diagonally. The analysis of the anatomic relationship of the A-P window shows that, even assuming the 10-mm gap, the real space for a biopsy narrows down to 5 mm when the tracheal wall is punctured at an angle of about 55° and is totally closed at an angle of about 42° (**Fig. 18**). So even with a needle that is long enough, biopsy of several nodes located in the middle and upper part of the A-P window area is not possible; the only way to them would lead through the aortic arch.

In conclusion, the station 5 and 6 nodes may be visualized using EUS, but the feasibility of needle biopsy is limited to the lower part of station 5 (see **Fig. 15C**) and is highly dependent on the actual anatomic relationships in the particular patient.

Learning Curve

There are no clear data regarding the number of EBUS or EUS procedures necessary for the endoscopist to gain enough experience and skill.

Block[42] presented the results of mediastinal staging in 4 periods: 10 months before introduction of EUS-NA, first 10 months of routine use of EUS-NA, first 8 months of using EUS-NA and EBUS-NA and the next 10 months. He concluded that the rate of unexpected N2 nodes discovered at surgery was higher initially, but in the subsequent periods it became comparable with those after mediastinoscopy.

In a prospective, multicenter study including data on 551 patients staged by EUS, Annema

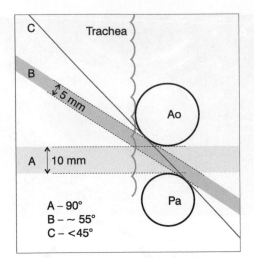

Fig. 18. Schematic drawing showing the gap between aortic arch and the left pulmonary artery, narrowing down as the angle between the needle tract and the tracheal wall is decreasing. Watching perpendicularly, the gap is 10 mm wide, but it narrows down to 5 mm when the angle of puncture is about 55° and closes totally at an angle of about 42°. The angle of transtracheal biopsy is 45° to 55°. Ao, aorta; Pa, left pulmonary artery.

and colleagues[43] showed different results. These investigators compared the diagnostic yield of EUS-NA performed by chest physicians in centers starting their EUS programs with those in an experienced expert center. There was no significant difference in sensitivity or accuracy of EUS-NA. Annema and colleagues concluded that endoscopists participating in a dedicated training program are able to achieve results similar to those of experts.

It seems necessary to develop evidence-based protocols for training in endosonographic techniques.[44]

Cost

Steinfort and colleagues[45] used decision-tree analysis to compare 4 strategies of invasive mediastinal staging, and found that the most cost-beneficial one was EBUS-NA with negative results being surgically confirmed (Australian dollars [A$] 2961) followed by EBUS-NA with negative results not surgically confirmed (A$3344), blind TBNA (A$3754), and mediastinoscopy, being almost 3 times more expensive than the first option (A$8859).

In another study, Harewood and colleagues[46] compared the cost of different staging methods. The cost (in US dollars) was lowest for EUS-NA ($11,490), followed by TBNA ($11,963),

PET ($12,887), CT-guided transthoracic biopsy ($13,027), and mediastinoscopy ($13,658).

Eight years later the same authors compared invasive staging modalities using a specially constructed decision model. These costs (in US dollars) were $18,603 for EUS-NA, $18,753 for CUS, $19,828 for EBUS-NA, $20,157 for mediastinoscopy, and $21,136 for TBNA.[47]

If the EUS as an initial staging procedure is compared with initial mediastinoscopy, the costs are $1867 and $12,900, respectively. The investigators concluded that using EUS-NA as the initial modality in patients with lung cancer reduces the number of mediastinoscopies by one-third.[48]

Comparison of the cost-effectiveness of EBUS-NA and mediastinoscopy was presented by Ang and colleagues[49] from Singapore, who showed that EBUS-NA results in the saving of 1214 Singapore dollars per positive staging.

A different strategy was adopted by Aabakken and colleagues,[50] who analyzed the cost of staging per year of expected survival. This cost was $1729 for EUS-NA and $2411 for mediastinoscopy.

In all of the cost-effectiveness analyses, the most cost-beneficial staging technique was EUS-NA or EBUS-NA. Mediastinoscopy, on the other hand, was consistently the most expensive method.

Box 1
Key Points

1. Endosonography-guided needle biopsy techniques enable the endoscopist to obtain adequate tissue specimens for cytologic or histologic assessment, which may be supplemented with immunohistochemical or genetic analysis

2. Both EBUS-NA and EUS-NA are safer and less expensive than surgical staging and use less hospital resources

3. The combination of ultrasonography with needle biopsy has a diagnostic yield superior to all other minimally invasive techniques and emerges as the most accurate option for mediastinal staging of lung cancer

4. In contrast to pulmonologists and gastroenterologists, thoracic surgeons are the most suitable for training in routine use of CUS, because they are accustomed to endoscopy of both the respiratory tract and the alimentary tract

5. In the near future, ongoing technical progress will expand the possibilities of endosonography even more

Complications

EBUS-NA and EUS-NA are safe procedures. Almost all published studies report no complications.[4,15,16,24,26,28–30,35,51,52] In a meta-analysis including 1201 patients who underwent EUS-NA, there were only 10 minor complications (0.8%).

There have been few case reports on the complications of endosonography-guided needle biopsy of mediastinal lymph nodes. Bauwens[53] described a case of pneumothorax in a patient with chronic obstructive pulmonary disease (COPD) who underwent EBUS-NA. In 1 patient with COPD a self-limiting hypoxemia was noted during EBUS-NA,[54] and in another a small (<30 mL) hemorrhage was observed.[55] Two cases of infectious complications after EBUS-NA with full needle length tissue penetration were reported. One of these patients developed bacterial pericarditis and the second developed infection of the tumor bed.[56]

SUMMARY

A review of the current literature clearly shows several aspects of endosonography-guided needle biopsy of mediastinal lymph nodes, which are outlined in **Box 1**.

REFERENCES

1. Hurtgen M, Friedel G, Toomes H, et al. Radical video-assisted mediastinoscopic lymphadenectomy (VAMLA)—technique and first results. Eur J Cardiothorac Surg 2002;21:348–51.
2. Kuzdzal J, Zielinski M, Papla B, et al. Transcervical extended mediastinal lymphadenectomy—the new operative technique and early results in lung cancer staging. Eur J Cardiothorac Surg 2005;27:384–90 [discussion: 90].
3. Kuzdzal J, Szlubowski A, Grochowski Z, et al. Current evidence on transcervical mediastinal lymph nodes dissection. Eur J Cardiothorac Surg 2011;40(6):1470–3.
4. Ye T, Hu H, Luo X, et al. The role of endobronchial ultrasound guided transbronchial needle aspiration (EBUS-TBNA) for qualitative diagnosis of mediastinal and hilar lymphadenopathy: a prospective analysis. BMC Cancer 2011;11:100.
5. Eloubeidi MA, Tamhane A, Jhala N, et al. Agreement between rapid onsite and final cytologic interpretations of EUS-guided FNA specimens: implications for the endosonographer and patient management. Am J Gastroenterol 2006;101:2841–7.
6. Wallace WA, Rassl DM. Accuracy of cell typing in non-small cell lung cancer by EBUS/EUS-FNA cytology samples. Eur Respir J 2011;38(4):911–7.
7. Nakajima T, Yasufuku K, Nakagawara A, et al. Multi-gene mutation analysis of metastatic lymph nodes in non-small cell lung cancer diagnosed by EBUS-TBNA. Chest 2011;140(5):1319–24.
8. Billah S, Stewart J, Staerkel G, et al. EGFR and KRAS mutations in lung carcinoma: molecular testing by using cytology specimens. Cancer Cytopathol 2011;119:111–7.
9. van Eijk R, Licht J, Schrumpf M, et al. Rapid KRAS, EGFR, BRAF and PIK3CA mutation analysis of fine needle aspirates from non-small-cell lung cancer using allele-specific qPCR. PLoS One 2011;6: e17791.
10. Schuurbiers OC, Looijen-Salamon MG, Ligtenberg MJ, et al. A brief retrospective report on the feasibility of epidermal growth factor receptor and KRAS mutation analysis in transesophageal ultrasound- and endobronchial ultrasound-guided fine needle cytological aspirates. J Thorac Oncol 2010;5:1664–7.
11. Garcia-Olive I, Monso E, Andreo F, et al. Endobronchial ultrasound-guided transbronchial needle aspiration for identifying EGFR mutations. Eur Respir J 2010;35:391–5.
12. Nakajima T, Yasufuku K, Suzuki M, et al. Assessment of epidermal growth factor receptor mutation by endobronchial ultrasound-guided transbronchial needle aspiration. Chest 2007;132:597–602.
13. Sakairi Y, Nakajima T, Yasufuku K, et al. EML4-ALK fusion gene assessment using metastatic lymph node samples obtained by endobronchial ultrasound-guided transbronchial needle aspiration. Clin Cancer Res 2010;16:4938–45.
14. Vilmann P, Krasnik M, Larsen SS, et al. Transesophageal endoscopic ultrasound-guided fine-needle aspiration (EUS-FNA) and endobronchial ultrasound-guided transbronchial needle aspiration (EBUS-TBNA) biopsy: a combined approach in the evaluation of mediastinal lesions. Endoscopy 2005; 37:833–9.
15. Hwangbo B, Lee GK, Lee HS, et al. Transbronchial and transesophageal fine-needle aspiration using an ultrasound bronchoscope in mediastinal staging of potentially operable lung cancer. Chest 2010; 138:795–802.
16. Herth FJ, Krasnik M, Kahn N, et al. Combined endoscopic-endobronchial ultrasound-guided fine-needle aspiration of mediastinal lymph nodes through a single bronchoscope in 150 patients with suspected lung cancer. Chest 2010;138:790–4.
17. Szlubowski A, Soja J, Kocon P, et al. A comparison of the combined ultrasound of the mediastinum by use of a single ultrasound bronchoscope versus ultrasound bronchoscope plus ultrasound gastroscope in lung cancer staging—a prospective trial. Interact Cardiovasc Thorac Surg 2011;13:321.
18. Detterbeck FC, Jantz MA, Wallace M, et al. Invasive mediastinal staging of lung cancer: ACCP evidence-based clinical practice guidelines (2nd edition). Chest 2007;132:202S–20S.

19. Adams K, Shah PL, Edmonds L, et al. Test performance of endobronchial ultrasound and transbronchial needle aspiration biopsy for mediastinal staging in patients with lung cancer: systematic review and meta-analysis. Thorax 2009;64:757–62.

20. Feller-Kopman D, Yung RC, Burroughs F, et al. Cytology of endobronchial ultrasound-guided transbronchial needle aspiration: a retrospective study with histology correlation. Cancer 2009;117:482–90.

21. Gilbert S, Wilson DO, Christie NA, et al. Endobronchial ultrasound as a diagnostic tool in patients with mediastinal lymphadenopathy. Ann Thorac Surg 2009;88:896–900 [discussion: 1–2].

22. Ernst A, Eberhardt R, Krasnik M, et al. Efficacy of endobronchial ultrasound-guided transbronchial needle aspiration of hilar lymph nodes for diagnosing and staging cancer. J Thorac Oncol 2009;4:947–50.

23. Hwangbo B, Kim SK, Lee HS, et al. Application of endobronchial ultrasound-guided transbronchial needle aspiration following integrated PET/CT in mediastinal staging of potentially operable non-small cell lung cancer. Chest 2009;135:1280–7.

24. Szlubowski A, Kuzdzal J, Kolodziej M, et al. Endobronchial ultrasound-guided needle aspiration in the non-small cell lung cancer staging. Eur J Cardiothorac Surg 2009;35:332–5 [discussion: 5–6].

25. Rintoul RC, Tournoy KG, El Daly H, et al. EBUS-TBNA for the clarification of PET positive intra-thoracic lymph nodes-an international multi-centre experience. J Thorac Oncol 2009;4:44–8.

26. Omark Petersen H, Eckardt J, Hakami A, et al. The value of mediastinal staging with endobronchial ultrasound-guided transbronchial needle aspiration in patients with lung cancer. Eur J Cardiothorac Surg 2009;36:465–8.

27. Defranchi SA, Edell ES, Daniels CE, et al. Mediastinoscopy in patients with lung cancer and negative endobronchial ultrasound guided needle aspiration. Ann Thorac Surg 2010;90:1753–7.

28. Nguyen TQ, Kalade A, Prasad S, et al. Endoscopic ultrasound guided fine needle aspiration (EUS-FNA) of mediastinal lesions. ANZ J Surg 2011;81:75–8.

29. Talebian M, von Bartheld MB, Braun J, et al. EUS-FNA in the preoperative staging of non-small cell lung cancer. Lung Cancer 2010;69:60–5.

30. Annema JT, Versteegh MI, Veselic M, et al. Endoscopic ultrasound-guided fine-needle aspiration in the diagnosis and staging of lung cancer and its impact on surgical staging. J Clin Oncol 2005;23:8357–61.

31. Singh P, Camazine B, Jadhav Y, et al. Endoscopic ultrasound as a first test for diagnosis and staging of lung cancer: a prospective study. Am J Respir Crit Care Med 2007;175:345–54.

32. Witte B, Neumeister W, Huertgen M. Does endoesophageal ultrasound-guided fine-needle aspiration replace mediastinoscopy in mediastinal staging of thoracic malignancies? Eur J Cardiothorac Surg 2008;33:1124–8.

33. Storch I, Shah M, Thurer R, et al. Endoscopic ultrasound-guided fine-needle aspiration and Trucut biopsy in thoracic lesions: when tissue is the issue. Surg Endosc 2008;22:86–90.

34. Wallace MB, Pascual JM, Raimondo M, et al. Minimally invasive endoscopic staging of suspected lung cancer. JAMA 2008;299:540–6.

35. Szlubowski A, Zielinski M, Soja J, et al. A combined approach of endobronchial and endoscopic ultrasound-guided needle aspiration in the radiologically normal mediastinum in non-small-cell lung cancer staging–a prospective trial. Eur J Cardiothorac Surg 2010;37:1175–9.

36. Szlubowski A, Kuzdzal J, Soja J, et al. A combined approach of endobronchial and endoscopic ultrasound-guided needle aspiration in the non-small cell lung cancer staging–a prospective study. Am J Respir Crit Care Med 2009;179:A1112.

37. Szlubowski A, Herth FJ, Soja J, et al. Endobronchial ultrasound-guided needle aspiration in non-small-cell lung cancer restaging verified by the transcervical bilateral extended mediastinal lymphadenectomy–a prospective study. Eur J Cardiothorac Surg 2010;37:1180–4.

38. Herth FJ, Annema JT, Eberhardt R, et al. Endobronchial ultrasound with transbronchial needle aspiration for restaging the mediastinum in lung cancer. J Clin Oncol 2008;26:3346–50.

39. Fujiwara T, Yasufuku K, Nakajima T, et al. The utility of sonographic features during endobronchial ultrasound-guided transbronchial needle aspiration for lymph node staging in patients with lung cancer: a standard endobronchial ultrasound image classification system. Chest 2010;138:641–7.

40. Gill KR, Ghabril MS, Jamil LH, et al. Endosonographic features predictive of malignancy in mediastinal lymph nodes in patients with lung cancer. Gastrointest Endosc 2010;72:265–71.

41. Sawhney MS, Debold SM, Kratzke RA, et al. Central intranodal blood vessel: a new EUS sign described in mediastinal lymph nodes. Gastrointest Endosc 2007;65:602–8.

42. Block MI. Transition from mediastinoscopy to endoscopic ultrasound for lung cancer staging. Ann Thorac Surg 2010;89:885–90.

43. Annema JT, Bohoslavsky R, Burgers S, et al. Implementation of endoscopic ultrasound for lung cancer staging. Gastrointest Endosc 2010;71:64–70, e1.

44. Unroe MA, Shofer SL, Wahidi MM. Training for endobronchial ultrasound: methods for proper training in new bronchoscopic techniques. Curr Opin Pulm Med 2010;16:295–300.

45. Steinfort DP, Liew D, Conron M, et al. Cost-benefit of minimally invasive staging of non-small cell lung

cancer: a decision tree sensitivity analysis. J Thorac Oncol 2010;5:1564–70.

46. Harewood GC, Wiersema MJ, Edell ES, et al. Cost-minimization analysis of alternative diagnostic approaches in a modeled patient with non-small cell lung cancer and subcarinal lymphadenopathy. Mayo Clin Proc 2002;77:155–64.

47. Harewood GC, Pascual J, Raimondo M, et al. Economic analysis of combined endoscopic and endobronchial ultrasound in the evaluation of patients with suspected non-small cell lung cancer. Lung Cancer 2010;67:366–71.

48. Eloubeidi MA, Tamhane A, Chen VK, et al. Endoscopic ultrasound-guided fine-needle aspiration in patients with non-small cell lung cancer and prior negative mediastinoscopy. Ann Thorac Surg 2005; 80:1231–9.

49. Ang SY, Tan RW, Koh MS, et al. Economic analysis of endobronchial ultrasound (EBUS) as a tool in the diagnosis and staging of lung cancer in Singapore. Int J Technol Assess Health Care 2010;26:170–4.

50. Aabakken L, Silvestri GA, Hawes R, et al. Cost-efficacy of endoscopic ultrasonography with fine-needle aspiration vs. mediastinotomy in patients with lung cancer and suspected mediastinal adenopathy. Endoscopy 1999;31:707–11.

51. Herth FJ, Eberhardt R, Krasnik M, et al. Endobronchial ultrasound-guided transbronchial needle aspiration of lymph nodes in the radiologically and positron emission tomography—normal mediastinum in patients with lung cancer. Chest 2008;133: 887–91.

52. Vincent BD, El-Bayoumi E, Hoffman B, et al. Real-time endobronchial ultrasound-guided transbronchial lymph node aspiration. Ann Thorac Surg 2008;85:224–30.

53. Bauwens O, Dusart M, Pierard P, et al. Endobronchial ultrasound and value of PET for prediction of pathological results of mediastinal hot spots in lung cancer patients. Lung Cancer 2008;61:356–61.

54. Lee HS, Lee GK, Lee HS, et al. Real-time endobronchial ultrasound-guided transbronchial needle aspiration in mediastinal staging of non-small cell lung cancer: how many aspirations per target lymph node station? Chest 2008;134:368–74.

55. Kanoh K, Miyazawa T, Kurimoto N, et al. Endobronchial ultrasonography guidance for transbronchial needle aspiration using a double-channel bronchoscope. Chest 2005;128:388–93.

56. Haas AR. Infectious complications from full extension endobronchial ultrasound transbronchial needle aspiration. Eur Respir J 2009;33:935–8.

Sentinel Lymph Node in Lung Cancer Surgery

Franca M.A. Melfi, MD[a],*, Federico Davini, MD[a],
Giuseppe Boni, MD[b], Alfredo Mussi, MD[a]

KEYWORDS

- Robotic • Lobectomy • Lung cancer • Thoracic surgery
- Sentinel lymph node • Non small cell lung cancer
- Micrometastasis • Polymerase chain reaction

Lung cancer is one of the most common malignancies in the western world and accounts for more cancer deaths than the next 4 most frequent cancers combined.[1,2] The overall low 5-year survival rate for patients diagnosed with lung cancer (15%) is especially discouraging.

Complete surgical resection for localized disease is the most viable option for sustained remission or cure. Patients relapsing after complete resection of stage I tumors by definition had occult disseminated disease at the time of their initial surgery. Such poor long-term survival is probably because early-stage disease is asymptomatic and the onset of symptoms marks the presence of advanced and incurable disease.

Staging is the primary determinant of survival. The main goals are to assist in determining appropriate treatment options (surgical vs nonsurgical) and in predicting prognosis. Based on the recommendation of the American Joint Committee for Cancer (AJCC), a TNM (tumor, node, and metastases) staging system is used for non–small-cell lung cancer (NSCLC).[2,3]

Conventional clinical staging modalities include history and physical examination, laboratory tests, and noninvasive staging techniques, such as chest radiographs, computed tomography (CT), bone scan, magnetic resonance imaging, and positron emission tomography (PET). If these tests do not suggest the presence of metastatic disease or unresectable local disease, further invasive staging procedures, including bronchoscopy, mediastinoscopy, and video-assisted thoracoscopic surgery, may be required.

Adjunctive invasive N-staging modalities, such as complete thoracic lymphadenectomy or nodal sampling, may help to further stratify patients into appropriate therapeutic and prognostic categories.

Mediastinal lymph node dissection is also an effective therapeutic procedure when performed in patients with nodal metastatic NSCLC; indeed, the status of lymph node metastasis is an important prognostic indicator.[4,5] On the other hand, mediastinal lymph node dissection is not therapeutic and may even be harmful.

The role of complete mediastinal lymph node dissection versus sampling at the time of thoracotomy remains controversial. Advocates of complete lymphadenectomy believe that without complete resection of nodal tissue, residual cancer may remain, leading to poorer prognosis because of regional recurrence and understaging of disease.[6,7] Conversely, proponents of lymph node sampling argue that sampling does not impair local immune factors that may reduce the potential for local recurrence, and is not associated with increased morbidity.[8] To date, no survival advantage has been clearly demonstrated using either technique.

[a] Division of Thoracic Surgery, Cardiothoracic and Vascular Department, University of Pisa, Via paradisa\2, 56124 Pisa, Italy
[b] Regional Center of Nuclear Medicine, University of Pisa, Via Roma 4, 56124 Pisa, Italy
* Corresponding author.
E-mail address: franca_melfi@hotmail.com

Thorac Surg Clin 22 (2012) 205–214
doi:10.1016/j.thorsurg.2011.12.008
1547-4127/12/$ – see front matter © 2012 Elsevier Inc. All rights reserved.

Whether to perform complete dissection or lymph node sampling at the time of lung cancer resection is a controversial subject. There is no dispute, however, regarding the prognostic importance of lymph node pathologic status. In patients with operable lung cancers, the presence of lymph node involvement may decrease the 5-year survival rate by nearly 50% as compared with similar patients without nodal metastases.[9,10]

If the prognosis of NSCLC is truly not affected by complete mediastinal lymph node dissection, it would be possible that morbidity of selective mediastinal lymph node sampling and pathologic staging of lung cancer can be improved by sentinel lymph node (SLN) mapping.

The prognosis of patients with NSCLC is closely related to the pathologic stage of the disease, with the pattern of regional lymph node (LN) involvement as a major determinant.[11] Although surgical treatment represents the best chance in 30% of patients with early-stage cancer, a high relapse rate (40%) is recorded within 24 months after complete resection (surgery and complete lymphadenectomy).[12–14] Undetected metastatic disease is the cause of these recurrences, which may remain undetected for 3 reasons[11]: inadequacy of lymphadenectomy (the lymph nodes draining the tumor are either not removed or incompletely removed),[12] inadequacy of pathologic examinations (methods used to detect tumor-derived material in LNs are insensitive), and the lymphatic drainage does not always follow the predicted pattern.[13]

Previous studies sought to improve identification of LN micrometastases during surgery through SLN mapping, or to improve the sensitivity of detecting tumor cells within the resection. Experience with melanoma[15] and breast cancer[16] demonstrated that SLNs were diagnostically accurate in predicting the status of more distant lymph node stations.

In NSCLC, a few studies identified SLN in more than 80% of patients and the SLN status was predictive in 80% to 100% of patients.[17–19] We previously reported the positive results achieved in detecting SLN with a ^{99m}Tc-nanocolloid suspension and micrometastasis by immunohistochemistry (IHC) in patients with stage I NSCLC[19]; however, these standard detection methods show low sensitivity. Reverse transcriptase-polymerase chain reaction (RT-PCR), which was developed to detect transcripts of genes expressed by tumor cells, is a tool for detecting LN-micrometastasis that is more sensitive than IHC.[20–22] Micrometastasis detected by RT-PCR has been associated with a worse prognosis in patients with melanoma and prostate carcinoma.[23–25] In lung cancer, few reports exist in this field[26,27]; however, published data has demonstrated how the molecular analysis could greatly improve the detection of micrometastases in patients with N0 disease.[3,19,28]

THE CONCEPT OF SENTINEL LYMPH NODE IN NSCLC

SLN is commonly defined as the first lymph node that receives afferent lymphatic drainage from a primary tumor. Several studies on the use of the SLN mapping in the treatment of NSCLC have been reported and they all show evidence of the existence of SLNs in NSCLC.[19,29–32]

The primary benefit of SLN mapping and biopsy is that it enables surgeons to avoid nontherapeutic lymph node dissection and the complications that follow. Nevertheless, the SLN concept is not yet approved as routine in clinical practice for patients with NSCLC.

SLN mapping and biopsy were developed as techniques for staging the lymphatic basin without the potential morbidity of lymphedema and nerve injury in cases of melanoma or lymphedema of the arm in cases of breast cancer. Lung resection for NSCLC with mediastinal lymph node dissection leads to a greater production of postoperative exudates than when compared with similar procedures performed without nodal dissection; however, morbidity related to mediastinal lymph node dissection is not significantly higher.

The most important utility of SLN mapping and biopsy is probably related to the ability to direct the pathologic examination to the first site of NSCLC nodal drainage, after which more sensitive techniques (IHC, serial sectioning, and RT-PCR analysis) can be applied to detect occult micrometastatic nodal disease.[30,33] Several groups have shown that more careful pathologic evaluation of previously reported negative lymph nodes in patients with resected lung cancer revealed that more than 20% of patients classified as having negative lymph nodes (N0) were actually upstaged by IHC with the identification of previously undetected micrometastatic disease.[34,35]

The ultrastaging made possible by sentinel node evaluation and the recognition of frequent mediastinal sentinel nodes may have a profound effect on the future staging of lung cancer. If confirmed by further studies, these results may lead to revisions of the TNM staging system, such as the inclusion of information related to the number of involved nodes and degree of nodal invasion. These findings form the basis of a multi-institutional trial designed to validate and refine the intraoperative sentinel node mapping technique.

SLN TECHNIQUES
Nonradionuclide Methods

Several techniques using nonradionuclide tracers for SLN mapping in patients with NSCLC have been proposed and developed.[29,35,36]

In 1999, Little and colleagues[29] first reported the intraoperative lymphatic mapping of the SLN in NSCLC using isosulfan blue. Unfortunately, the identification rate of the SLN was only 46%: too low to be clinically useful. Sugi and colleagues[35] reported a lower identification rate (6.3%) of the SLN with indocyanine green. Also, anaphylactic reactions to these dyes occurred, although rarely.[37]

More recently, Japanese investigators developed a novel method that uses the magnetic force.[36] As a tracer, colloidal ferumoxides (superparamagnetic iron) were injected during thoracotomy at the periphery of the tumor. A highly sensitive, handheld magnetometer was use to detect ex vivo the magnetic force of the ferumoxides within SLNs. The preliminary results seem to indicate that this approach is feasible and safe but not suitable for in vivo SLN mapping until now.

Finally, fluorescent-labeled agents, such as vitamin B12, have been tested in animals, but these agents will need to be further investigated before their use in humans.[38]

Radionuclide Methods

Liptay,[30] in 2000, first described the surgical technique of radioguided localization of SLN in NSCLC. At the time of thoracotomy, the tumor was injected in a 4-quadrant peritumoral fashion with 2 mCi of [99m]technetium sulfur colloid filtered once through a 20-μm filter. Then the operation proceeded normally, with care to avoid peribronchial lymphatics until the last part of the resection. Radioactive counting of both the primary tumor and lymph nodes was obtained with a hand-held gamma counter. Anatomic resection with formal mediastinal node dissection was performed and findings were correlated with histology. Sentinel nodes were defined as any nodal station with radioactivity readings 3 times greater than background measurements in the thorax. Multiple sentinel node stations were identified in approximately 15% of cases. Radioactive lymph nodes identified as SLNs were examined after staining with hematoxylin-eosin (H&E) and IHC with a cytokeratin antibody.

The migration mean time of the radiocolloids through the lymphatics was 63 minutes (range 23–170) and did not prolong the operation; no associated morbidities were identified. The SLN identification rate was 82%, and the false-negative rate was 5.4%. Three of 37 patients were upstaged

from N0 to N1 by IHC and serial section analysis of sentinel nodes. Liptay[30] also noted that 22% of the identified sentinel nodes were found to be mediastinal (N2) or had a "skip pattern" of nodal drainage, skipping over the more proximal lobar and hilar (N1) stations.

Liptay[30] concluded that the intraoperative technique was feasible and safe; however, discovered that this technique was unable to obtain useful radioactive signal from the upper mediastinal lymph node during surgery, owing to interfering background from the radiotracer that had migrated into the trachea from the lung. Therefore, Liptay[30] identified the mediastinal SLNs by ex vivo counting after mediastinal lymph node dissection.

To overcome this drawback, Liptay and colleagues[30] modified the original technique, decreasing the amount of radioactivity injected into the tumors from an original total dose of 2 mCi to our current dose of 0.25 mCi. This adjustment in technique has allowed a significant decrease in background radiation from the tumor, enhancing our ability to identify a unique SLN station in vivo.

Nomori and colleagues[31] first reported in 2002 the preoperative injection of 6 to 8 mCi of [99m]technetium tin colloid with a single shot into peritumoral regions using a CT-guided technique and then detected SLNs intraoperatively using a gamma probe. Subsequently, other groups[19,35] used the CT-guided preoperative injection technique, reporting an SLN identification rate (67%–87%) similar to that obtained by the intraoperative injection procedure of Liptay.

The most important advantage of the preoperative injection technique is that it enables intraoperative measurement of gamma counts in the upper mediastinal lymph node, because coughing by the patient rapidly removes radioisotope from the trachea.

A useful alternative to CT-guided injection of the radiocolloids seems to be the preoperative transbronchoscopic injection. Lardinois and colleagues[32] investigated the feasibility of preoperative bronchoscopic injection of radiolabeled technetium-99 m nanocolloid in a group of 20 patients with T1-3 N0-1 NSCLC and obtained an SLN identification rate of 95%. No complication related to the procedure was observed.

All these reports demonstrated the feasibility of both preoperative and intraoperative injection in identifying the first site of potential nodal metastases of NSCLC.

A number of investigators have reported that when using the radioisotope method, there is minimal exposure to radiation for surgeons, pathologists, or other medical staff.[39,40] The radiation risk for patients is also low when compared with that of numerous other medical procedures, as well as the radioactive risk of the waste.[40] Nevertheless, radioactive materials should always be handled with care.

THE AUTHORS' EXPERIENCE

Our previous study on intraoperative SLN mapping established the feasibility of this technique and was the basis of this progress report on the evolving utility of this technique in lung cancer staging.[9] In the last 22 patients, we combined the SLN mapping technique with molecular staging using cytokeratin (CK) 7 and 19, which are markers of epithelial cells. We hypothesized that the RT-PCR for RNA detection of CK7 and CK19 would accurately detect micrometastases and define an improvement of staging in patients with early lung cancer (stage I disease). The preliminary results show that this technique could allow identification of a subgroup of patients in which the use of RT-PCR could be applied on a well-focused target. This approach may be useful for histologically stratifying N0 patients into higher risk and lower risk groups.

Methods

From May 2001, 51 consecutive patients with NSCLC (stage IA–IB) were enrolled. The first 29 were included in the first step of our study (validation phase). All resected lymph nodes were analyzed by conventional pathologic methods (H&E and IHC). The last 22 patients (11 female; median age 69 years, range: 56–78) were selected for SLN mapping by using a new protocol. SLNs were analyzed in 16 of 19 patients by using conventional pathologic examination (H&E/IHC), and molecular analysis by RT-PCR. The study was approved by the local ethics committee and informed consent was obtained from each patient.

Only patients able to tolerate anatomic resection and complete mediastinal node dissection were included in this study. Routine preoperative workup was performed, including clinical examination, blood chemistry analysis, chest x-ray, thoracic CT and PET scanning, abdominal ultrasonography, and bronchoscopy. Furthermore, bone scintigraphy and brain CT scan were performed in patients with suspected distant metastases. The tumor stage was classified according to the Revisions in the International System for Staging Lung Cancer.[3]

Selection criteria were (1) older than 18 years (legal majority), (2) clinical stage I NSCLC (stage IA–IB), and (3) absence of intrathoracic adenopathy with normal bronchoscopic appearance. Patients with pulmonary metastasis, previous thoracic surgery/adjuvant therapy, enlarged mediastinal lymph nodes more than 1 cm in short-axis diameter on CT/PET scan or with primary tumor larger than 3 cm were excluded. In accordance with our normal practice for small lesions without mediastinal lymphadenopathy (on the CT/PET scan), mediastinoscopy was not performed. These patients were considered at clinical stage I. Standard lobectomy combined with systematic lymph node dissection was performed to achieve complete anatomic resection of the tumor.

Technique

The SLN technique previously described in our article was similar to that of other investigators.[7–9] ^{99m}Tc-nanocolloids of human albumin (more than 95% with particle size <80 nm) was used. A total dose of 37 MBq in a maximum volume of 1 mL was administered in 2 to 4 divided aliquots (depending on the size of the tumor) injected at the periphery of the tumor. Readings were taken with the gamma ray detector (Scinti Probe MR100-Pol.hi.tech., Aquila, Italy) (**Fig. 1**). The radiotracer was administered on the basis of the tumor's location: tumors located close to the hilum were injected by bronchoscopy or at the time of thoracotomy; those located at periphery were injected under CT guidance or by thoracoscopy. The molecular analysis (RT-PCR) was added at conventional pathologic SLN examination (H&E and IHC).

Peripheral tumors

These tumors were localized by means of 5-mm-thick high-resolution axial CT sections or by 7-mm endoscopic camera usually at the sixth/seventh intercostal space along the midaxillary line. A 22-G needle was introduced at the peripheral margins of the tumor through which the radiotracer was injected.

Central tumors

The radioisotope suspension was administered by a fiberoptic bronchoscope or directly during thoracotomy if bronchoscopic injection was not feasible. This procedure was performed under fluoroscopic guidance by using an endoscopic needle inserted at the carina of the most distal pulmonary subsegment close to the tumor (**Fig. 2**).

The intraoperative radioactivity counting at the nodal stations started an average of 1 hour (range 50–70 minutes) after the injection. The radiolabeled tumor and lymph node stations were examined in vivo and ex vivo. The migration of the ^{99m}Tc-nanocolloid suspension was considered successful if a specific nodal station measured greater than 3 times the background. The sentinel node was classified as the node(s) with the highest count rate.

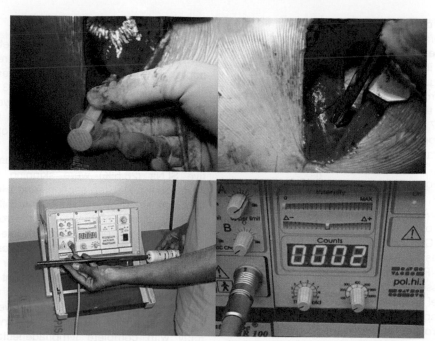

Fig. 1. Intraoperative injection and handheld sterile-draped Gamma counter. (*Courtesy of* Scinti Probe MR 100-Pol.hi.tech., Aquila, Italy; with permission.)

At the end of the operation (after lobectomy and excision of the sentinel lymph node) the mediastinal stations were also examined before performing a complete lymph node dissection. On completion of the procedure, a repeated examination with gamma probe was performed to check residual activity. If indicated by the gamma counter, we completed re-resections of the nodal stations.

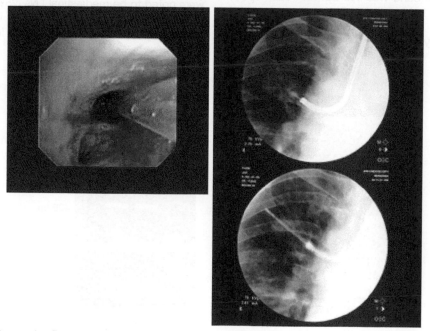

Fig. 2. Injection under fluoroscopic guidance by using an endoscopic-needle inserted at the carina of the most distal pulmonary subsegment close to the tumor. (*From* Melfi FM, Lucchi M, Davini F, et al. Intraoperative sentinel lymph node mapping in stage I non-small cell lung cancer: detection of micrometastases by polymerase chain reaction. Eur J Cardiothorac Surg 2008;34:181–6; with permission.)

Pathologic details

No intraoperative frozen sections were performed. Half of the SLN was fixed in formalin and embedded in paraffin for histologic analysis and IHC staining. The other half of the resected node was snap-frozen in liquid nitrogen and stored at −80°C until the time of RNA isolation for the analysis of CK7 and CK19, as markers of epithelial differentiation. After formalin fixation and embedding in paraffin, sections (2 or 3) were cut and stained with H&E. Sentinel and nonsentinel nodes were subsequently examined by IHC for pankeratin CK, CK7, and CK19 (Ventana Medical System, Inc, AZ, USA). Molecular analysis (RT-PCR) was applied in our second series. The presence of mRNA for CK7 and CK19 within the SLNs was accepted as evidence of micrometastatic tumor cells. The RNA was extracted by a standard method, assessed by electrophoresis on a 0.8% agarose gel to determine its integrity, and was quantified spectrophotometrically (**Fig. 3**).

Using 2 rounds of amplifications (RT-PCR) and serial dilutions of RNA, it was possible to detect down to 1 tumoral cell in 10^6. The cycling conditions were as follows: 94°C for 1 minute, 68°C for 2 minutes for 20 cycles for the first PCR and 20 cycles for the second PCR. All PCR reactions were preceded by a denaturation step at 94°C for 3 minutes, and terminated by a 10-minute extension at 72°C. The expected size for CK19 amplification band was 409 bp. All frozen specimens were held until the final pathology report was issued in case the tissue was needed for routine analysis.

RESULTS

Positive results in detecting micrometastasis (by IHC) in the first series (29 patients) were previously published.[19] In the first study, SLNs were identified in 96.1% of patients, with a total of 31 SLNs detected. Seven (22.5%) of 31 SLNs were positive for metastatic involvement after full histopathologic evaluation (including IHC). In 2 of 7 of these positive SLNs (positive SLN in level 10) IHC revealed an additional positive N2 station. Two positive SLNs (28.5%) were skipping metastases (levels 9 and 7). Step sections and IHC examination revealed micrometastases in 5 (20%) of 25 patients without metastasis in the routine H&E-stained sections. Overall Kaplan-Meier survival at 3 years was 78.1 ± 11 months for p-stage I patients versus 50 ± 12.3 months for overstaged patients (with IHC). No significant difference (P = .1) was observed.

In the second series, 22 patients were selected for SLN mapping. All patients underwent lobectomy with complete lymphadenectomy. SLNs were detected in 16 of 19 patients. In 3 of the 19 patients (#17, #18, #19) SLNs were not identified because of incorrect technique in which the radiotracer injected into the tumor had poor migration because the tracer was not administered at the periphery.

A single SLN was identified in each patient (total number of SLNs were 16). Among the 16 SLNs, 5 were noted to be mediastinal LNs (25%), of which 2 were level 7 and 2 were level 4; 1 was level 8. Five SLNs were found at level 10, 4 at level 11, and

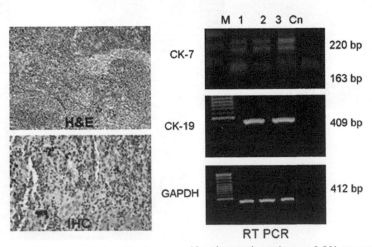

Fig. 3. The RNA extracted by a standard method, assessed by electrophoresis on a 0.8% agarose gel to determine its integrity and was quantified spectrophotometrically. (*From* Melfi FM, Lucchi M, Davini F, et al. Intraoperative sentinel lymph node mapping in stage I non-small cell lung cancer: detection of micrometastases by polymerase chain reaction. Eur J Cardiothorac Surg 2008;34:181–6; with permission.)

2 at level 12. H&E revealed 15 adenocarcinomas, 2 squamous cell carcinomas, 1 large-cell carcinoma, and 1 bronchoalveolar carcinoma. According to the TNM classification, pathologic staging identified 10 patients with stage I disease, 1 patient with stage IIB, 4 patients with stage IIIA disease, and 1 patient with stage IIIB disease. IHC examination had micrometastases in 7 (43.75%) of 16 patients; 2 of them were evaluated as N0 by H&E staining. RT-PCR analysis was applied in 10 of 16 patients (in the remaining 6 samples, the frozen half of each SLN was insufficient). Micrometastases were detected in 6 patients; 4 of these evaluated as N0 according to conventional examination (3 N0 by H&E, 1 N0 by IHC).

All SLNs tested by RT-PCR were also analyzed by H&E and IHC (**Fig. 4**). In 9 of 10 patients, RT-PCR confirmed the IHC staging in all SLNs that could be evaluated. Three patients (#9, #14, #15), who had stage I disease according to routine pathologic examination, were upstaged from stage I to stage II (from N0 to N1). Two of them (#9, #15) with positive IHC for pankeratin were also evaluated as stage II by RT-PCR. In the third patient (#14) with negative IHC, micrometastases were identified only by RT-PCR analysis. The presence of CK19 as a marker of epithelial differentiation was accepted as evidence of micrometastatis (see **Fig. 4**). This patient had a systemic relapse 3 months after surgery and died 4 months later. Any patients with N0 or N1 disease by RT-PCR staging had recurrences. Of the 5 patients with N2 disease according to the RT-PCR analysis, 3 (#1, #4, #8) patients developed recurrent disease 3, 13, and 14 months after surgery, respectively.

During the follow-up of 9 to 24 months, 3 patients died (#1, #8, #14) because of recurrent disease. Of the patients who remained alive, 1 patient with N2 disease (#4) has recurrence.

COMMENT

Lymph node metastasis is the most important prognostic factor in localized and resectable NSCLC. Patients with N0 disease have favorable survival rates; however, up to 40% of these patients have a recurrence of the tumor and subsequently die, despite complete surgical resection.[34] This suggests that occult micrometastases, undetected at preoperative staging and with routine histopathologic methods, have already spread to the regional nodes at the time of surgery.[1–4] Therefore, a plausible explanation could be inadequate nodal dissection or inadequate pathologic analysis.[35,36]

SLN is commonly defined as the first lymph node that receives afferent lymphatic drainage from a primary tumor[5–11]; therefore, this node is the first site of lymphatic involvement if metastasis has occurred. If this concept is correct, when metastasis is not found in an SLN, it most likely will not be present in the more distal nodes. As shown for early stages in malignant melanoma and breast cancer, the SLN allowed selective sensitive pathologic analysis to assess micrometastases.[5,6] In NSCLC, a few studies identified SLNs in more than 80% of patients, and found that the SLN status was predictive of the status of all other LNs in 80% to 100% of patients[5,41,42]; however, standard detection methods have a low sensitivity. Better methods for detecting SLN involvement would improve the ability to determine the risk of recurrence, which may affect patient treatment. The staining of serial sections of SLNs by IHC has been the most reported method of identifying micrometastases.

Molecular analysis of CK 7 and 19 by RT-PCR offers a sensitive tool for the detection of micrometastasis[10–12]; however, this takes advantage of the development of a variety of probes for genes that may be overexpressed in certain tumors. For melanoma, this includes tyrosinase-related proteins (TRP-1, TRP-2), microphthalmia-associated transcription factor, MAGE-3, gp100, and MART-1; for breast cancer, CK 19, 12 MUC-1, 13 mammaglobin B, 14 and MAGE-A3 15 have been identified as potential markers, among others. Carcinoembryonic antigen and MAGE-A are the most frequently used in colon cancer.[43]

Few studies exist in lung cancer.[26] Our preliminary data found RT-PCR evidence of micrometastasis in

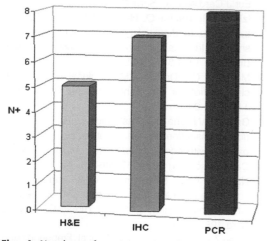

Lymph node metastasis identification rate

Fig. 4. Number of positive SLNs by each method. (*From* Melfi FM, Lucchi M, Davini F, et al. Intraoperative sentinel lymph node mapping in stage I non-small cell lung cancer: detection of micrometastases by polymerase chain reaction. Eur J Cardiothorac Surg 2008;34:181–6; with permission.)

6 of 10 SLNs that could be evaluated. An interesting result was the presence of CK19 as a marker of epithelial differentiation in 1 patient (#14) who was evaluated as N0 by IHC, and who was upstaged from stage I (T1N0) to stage II (T1N1) only by molecular analysis. In this case, the presence of CK was accepted as evidence of micrometastasis; however, because the prognostic significance of molecular upstaging in NSCLC is not yet known, this patient was considered as stage IA, and thus no adjuvant chemotherapy was administered. On the other hand, although adjuvant chemotherapy is becoming the standard of care for most patients with NSCLC, and recent studies have demonstrated its benefits in early staging,[44] the real advantage in patients with lung cancer remains unclear. Intraoperative SLN mapping in this field could be useful for stratifying histologically N0 patients into higher-risk groups.

Regarding the role of radical lymphadenectomy in patients with stage I lung cancer (especially those who underwent SLN mapping), it is still considered a critical point. Some randomized trials (Izbicki and colleagues[14]) showed no survival benefit; others stressed the therapeutic value of radical systematic lymphadenectomy.[45,46]

SLN biopsy was initially developed as a minimally invasive surgical alternative to routine (elective) complete lymphadenectomy; however, lymphadenectomy for staging and therapeutic benefit in lung cancer still remains the gold standard for lung cancer staging. Taking all of this into consideration, we hypothesized that SLN mapping in lung cancer should be used to improve staging in patients with stage I disease. Therefore, in contrast with other solid tumors, in which this technique has been applied to minimize lymphadenectomy, in lung cancer this method should be considered as a new technique for stratifying N0 patients. This approach could be a useful way to enable pathologists to identify with higher sensitivity, micrometastasis. In conclusion, the current study confirmed the feasibility of SLN mapping in NSCLC, and demonstrated that SLN molecular studies could greatly improve the detection of micrometastases in patients with N0 disease. Thus, with increased experience, this technique may become a standard practice in the management of early-stage NSCLC. Just as micrometastases are codified as N0 substages in breast and colon cancers (AJCC staging systems),[45] a similar substage could be applied in patients with stage I lung cancer. The actual clinical impact of SLN mapping in lung cancer remains to be elucidated through further studies; moreover, molecular analysis needs to be performed largely in research settings (because the prognostic significance of positive RT-PCR is still unclear). Nevertheless, in the near future, this technique may be useful in selecting a subset of patients with NSCLC N0 who are most likely to be cured by surgery alone, as well as those patients who are more likely to benefit from adjuvant therapy.

REFERENCES

1. Jemal A, Siegel R, Ward E. Cancer Statistics, 2006. CA Cancer J Clin 2006;56:106–30.
2. Jemal RC, Tiwari T, Murray A, et al. Cancer Statistics, 2004. CA Cancer J Clin 2004;54:8–29.
3. Mountain CF. Revisions in the international system for staging lung cancer. Chest 1997;111:1710–7.
4. Nesbitt JC, Putnam JB, Walsh GL, et al. Survival in early-stage non-small cell lung cancer. Ann Thorac Surg 1995;60:466–72.
5. Keller SM, Adak S, Wagner H, et al. Mediastinal lymph node dissection improves survival in patients with stages II and IIIa non-small cell lung cancer. Eastern Cooperative Oncology Group. Ann Thorac Surg 2000;70:358–65 [discussion: 365–6].
6. Naruke T, Goya T, Tsuchiya R, et al. The importance of surgery to non-small cell carcinoma of lung with mediastinal lymph node metastasis. Ann Thorac Surg 1988;46:603–10.
7. Passlick B, Kubuschock B, Sienel W, et al. Mediastinal lymphadenectomy in non-small cell lung cancer: effectiveness in patients with or without nodal micrometastases—results of a preliminary study. Eur J Cardiothorac Surg 2002;21:520–6.
8. Naruke T, Tsuchiya R, Kondo H, et al. Lymph node sampling in lung cancer: how should it be done? Eur J Cardiothorac Surg 1999;16:17–24.
9. Izbicki JR, Thetter O, Habekost M, et al. Radical systematic mediastinal lymphadenectomy in non-small cell lung cancer: a randomized controlled trial. Br J Surg 1994;81:229–35.
10. Mountain CF, Dresler CM. Regional lymph node classification for lung cancer staging. Chest 1997;111:1718–23.
11. Graham AN, Chan KJ, Pastorino U, et al. Systematic nodal dissection in the intrathoracic staging of patients with non-small cell lung cancer. J Thorac Cardiovasc Surg 1999;117:246–51.
12. Naruke T, Goya T, Tsuchiya R, et al. Prognosis and survival in resected lung cancer based on the new international staging system. J Thorac Cardiovasc Surg 1988;96:440–7.
13. Chen Z-L, Perez S, Holmes EC, et al. Frequency and distribution of occult micrometastases in lymph nodes of patients with non-small cell lung carcinoma. J Natl Cancer Inst 1993;85:4493–8.
14. Izbicki JR, Passlick B, Hosch SB, et al. Mode of spread in the early phase of lymphatic metastases

in non-small cell lung cancer: significance of nodal micrometastases. J Thorac Cardiovasc Surg 1996; 112:623–30.

15. Morton DL, Duan-Ren W, Wong SG. Technical details of intraoperative lymphatic mapping for early stage melanoma. Arch Surg 1992;127:392–9.

16. Giuliano AE, Kirgan DM, Guentha JM, et al. Lymphatic mapping and sentinel lymphadenectomy for breast cancer. Ann Surg 1994;220:391–401.

17. Liptay MJ, Grodin SC, Winchester DJ, et al. Intraoperative radioisotope sentinel lymph node mapping in non-small cell lung cancer. Ann Thorac Surg 2000;70:384–9.

18. Nomori H, Horio H, Naruke T, et al. Use of thecnetium-99 m tin colloid for sentinel lymph node identification in NSCLC. J Thorac Cardiovasc Surg 2002;124:486–92.

19. Melfi FM, Chella A, Menconi GF, et al. Intraoperative radioguided sentinel lymph node biopsy in non-small cell lung cancer. Eur J Cardiothorac Surg 2003;23:214–20.

20. Blaheta HJ, Shittek B, Breuningen H. Detection of melanoma micrometastasis in sentinel nodes by reverse transcription polymerase chain reaction correlates with tumor thickness and is predictive of micrometastatic disease in the lymph node basin. Am J Surg Pathol 1999;23:822–8.

21. Deghuci T, Doi T, Ehara H, et al. Detection of micrometastatic prostate cancer cells in lymph nodes by reverse transcriptase polymerase chain reaction. Cancer Res 1993;53:5320–54.

22. Sanchez-Cespedes M, Esteller M, Hibi K, et al. Molecular detection of neoplastic cells in lymph nodes of metastatic colorectal cancer patients predicts recurrence. Clin Cancer Res 1999;5: 2450–4.

23. Shariat SF, Roudier MP, Wilcox GE, et al. Comparison of immunohistochemistry with reverse transcription PCR for the detection of micrometastatic prostate cancer in lymph nodes. Cancer Res 2003; 63:4662–70.

24. Blaheta HJ, Ellwanger U, Schittek B, et al. Examination of regional lymph nodes by sentinel node biopsy and molecular analysis provides new staging facilities in primary cutaneous melanoma. J Invest Dermatol 2000;114:637–42.

25. Okegawa T, Nutahara K, Higashihara E. Detection of micrometastatic prostate cancer cells in the lymph nodes by reverse transcriptase polymerase chain reaction is predictive of biochemical recurrence in pathological stage T2 prostate cancer. J Urol 2000; 163:1183–8.

26. Pulte D, Li E, Crawford BK, et al. Sentinel lymph node mapping and molecular staging in NSCLC. Cancer 2005;104:1453–61.

27. Strauss GM, Kwiatkawski DJ, Harpole DH, et al. Molecular and pathologic markers in stage I non-small cell carcinoma of the lung. J Clin Oncol 1995;13(5):1265–79.

28. Melfi FM, Lucchi M, Davini F, et al. Intraoperative sentinel lymph node mapping in stage I non small cell lung cancer: detection of micrometastases by polymerase chain reaction. Eur J Cardiothorac Surg 2008;34:181–6.

29. Little AG, DeHoyos A, Kirgan DM, et al. Intraoperative lymphatic mapping for non-small cell lung cancer: the sentinel node technique. J Thorac Cardiovasc Surg 1999;117:220–34.

30. Liptay MJ. Sentinel node mapping in lung cancer: the holy grail? Ann Thorac Surg 2008;85:S778–9.

31. Nomori H, Watanabe K, Ohtsuka T, et al. In vivo identification of sentinel lymph nodes for clinical stage I non-small cell lung cancer for abbreviation of mediastinal lymph node dissection. Lung Cancer 2004;46:49–55.

32. Lardinois D, Brack T, Gaspert A, et al. Bronchoscopic radioisotope injection for sentinel lymph-node mapping in potentially resectable non-small-cell lung cancer. Eur J Cardiothorac Surg 2003;23: 824–7.

33. Kubuschock B, Passlick B, Izbicki JR, et al. Disseminated tumor cells in lymph nodes as a determinant for survival in surgically resected non-small cell lung cancer. J Clin Oncol 1999;17:19–24.

34. Riquet M, Manac'h D, Pimpec-Barthes F, et al. Prognostic significance of surgical-pathologic N1 disease in non-small cell carcinoma of the lung. Ann Thorac Surg 1999;67:1572–6.

35. Sugi K, Fukuda M, Nakamura H, et al. Comparison of three tracers for detecting sentinel lymph nodes in patients with clinical N0 lung cancer. Lung Cancer 2003;39:37–40.

36. Nakagawa T, Minamiya Y, Katayose Y, et al. A novel method for sentinel lymph node mapping using magnetite in patients with non-small cell lung cancer. J Thorac Cardiovasc Surg 2003;126:563–7.

37. Albo D, Wayne JD, Hunt KK, et al. Anaphylactic reactions to isosulfan blue dye during sentinel lymph node biopsy for breast cancer. Am J Surg 2001;182: 393–8.

38. McGreevy JM, Cannon MJ, Grissom CB. Minimally invasive lymphatic mapping using fluorescently labeled vitamin B12. J Surg Res 2003;111:38–44.

39. Motta C, Turra A, Farina B, et al. Radioguided surgery of breast cancer: radiation protection survey. Tumori 2000;86:372–4.

40. Waddington WA, Keshtgar MR, Taylor I, et al. Radiation safety of the sentinel lymph node technique in breast cancer. Eur J Nucl Med 2000;27: 377–91.

41. Naruke T, Tsuchia R, Kondo H, et al. Implications of staging in lung cancer. Chest 1997;112:242S–8S.

42. Naruke T, Tsuchia R, Kondo H, et al. Prognosis and survival after resection for bronchogenic carcinoma

based on the 1997 TNM staging classification: the Japanese experience. Ann Thorac Surg 2001;71: 1759–64.

43. Greenson JK, Isenhart CE, Rice R, et al. Identification of occult micro metastases in pericolic lymph nodes of Duke's B colorectal cancer patients using monoclonal antibodies against cytokeratin and CC49. Correlation with long-term survival. Cancer 1994;73:563–9.

44. Strauss GM, Herndon J, Maddaus MA. Randomized clinical trial of adjuvant chemotherapy with paclitaxel and carboplatin following resection in stage IB NSCLC: report of Cancer and Leukemia Group B (CALGB) Protocol 9633. J Clin Oncol 2004; 22(Suppl 14):A7019.

45. Izbicki JR, Passlick B, Pantel K, et al. Effectiveness of radical systematic mediastinal lymphadenectomy in patients with resectable non-small cell lung cancer: results of a prospective randomized trial. Ann Surg 1998;227:138–44.

46. Martini N, Flehinger BJ, Zaman MB, et al. Results of resection in non-oat cell carcinoma of the lung with mediastinal lymph node metastases. Ann Surg 1983;198:386–97.

Thoracoscopic and Robotic Dissection of Mediastinal Lymph Nodes

Douglas J. Minnich, MD[a], Ayesha S. Bryant, MD, MSPH[b],
Robert J. Cerfolio, MD[c],*

KEYWORDS

- Mediastinum • Lymphadenectomy • Thoracoscopy
- Robotics

The mediastinum is an anatomic space that contains many lymphatic channels and lymph nodes. An appropriate understanding of this anatomy is relevant to many disease processes as well as therapeutic intervention for thoracic malignancies. A brief review of the anatomy of the mediastinal lymph nodes is precesnted and the indications for mediastinal lymph node dissection are discussed, followed by a more detailed description of the technical aspects of thoracoscopic and robotic mediastinal lymph node dissection.

ANATOMY

The lymph nodes of the mediastinum are organized by anatomic regions or stations, and are assigned a number that corresponds to that anatomic level.[1] The numbering was designed to allow surgeons to communicate with one another and to minimize confusion.

As shown in **Fig. 1**, the paratracheal spaces are numbered level 2 for high paratracheal space and level 4 for low paratracheal space. The aortopulmonary window is numbered level 5, whereas the region anterior to the arch of the aorta is assigned level 6. The subcarinal space is level 7. Lymph nodes in the paraesophageal region are level 8 and those within the inferior pulmonary ligament are level 9. For the paratracheal, paraesophageal, and inferior pulmonary ligament locations, a corresponding "R" is added for right-sided or an "L" for left-sided. These anatomic levels are depicted in **Fig. 1**. The only station that is midline and is not given a right or left designation is the subcarinal space (level 7). A right-sided mediastinal lymph node dissection should include the right paratracheal (levels 2R and 4R), subcarinal (level 7), paraesophageal (level 8), and the inferior pulmonary ligament (level 9). A left-sided mediastinal lymph node dissection should include the aortopulmonary window (level 5), anterior aortic (level 6), subcarinal (level 7), paraesophageal (level 8), and the inferior pulmonary ligament (level 9). The proximity of the carotid and subclavian arteries as well as the position of the left recurrent laryngeal nerve make it more difficult to remove the 4L and 5 lymph nodes, but the nodes should be completely removed despite these important structures.

This manuscript was not supported by any grant support.
Financial disclosures: Intuitive, Precision, Covidien (R.J.C); superDimension, Inc (D.J.M); None (A.S.B.).
[a] Division of Cardiothoracic Surgery, University of Alabama at Birmingham, 703 19th Street South, 716 ZRB, Birmingham, AL 35294, USA
[b] Division of Cardiothoracic Surgery, University of Alabama at Birmingham, 703 19th Street South, 736 ZRB, Birmingham, AL 35294, USA
[c] Division of Cardiothoracic Surgery, University of Alabama at Birmingham, 703 19th Street South, 739 ZRB, Birmingham, AL 35294, USA
* Corresponding author.
E-mail address: rcerfolio@uab.edu

Thorac Surg Clin 22 (2012) 215–218
doi:10.1016/j.thorsurg.2011.12.007
1547-4127/12/$ – see front matter

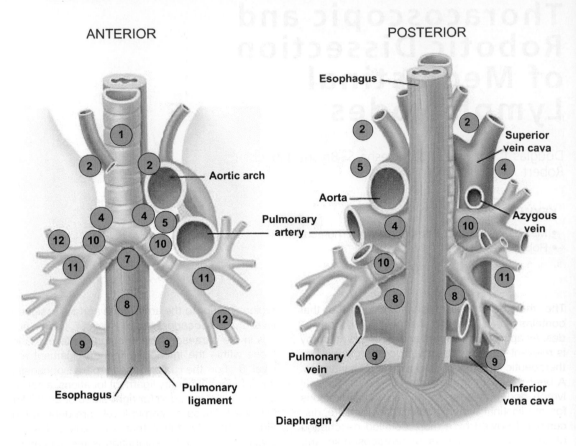

ANTERIOR

POSTERIOR

Esophagus

Aortic arch

Pulmonary artery

Superior vein cava

Aorta

Azygous vein

Pulmonary vein

Esophagus

Pulmonary ligament

Diaphragm

Inferior vena cava

Lymph Node Stations

Lymph Node Stations	Accessible by:
1 = Supraclavicular	EBUS-TBNA
2 = Upper paratracheal	EBUS-TBNA, Mediastinoscopy
3 = Prevascular	EBUS-TBNA, Mediastinoscopy
4 = Lower paratracheal	EBUS-TBNA, EUS-FNA, Mediastinoscopy
5 = Subaortic	VATS, EUS-FNA
6 = AP window (not shown)	VATS
7 = Subcarinal	EBUS-TBNA, EUS-FNA, Mediastinoscopy
8 = Paraesophageal	EBUS-TBNA, EUS-FNA
9 = Pulmonary ligament	EUS-FNA
10 = Hilar	EBUS-TBNA
11 = Interlobar	EBUS-TBNA
12 = Lobar	EBUS-TBNA

EBUS-TBNA = Endobronchial ultrasound guided transbronchial needle aspiration
EUS-FNA = Endoscopic ultrasound guided fine needle aspiration
VATS = Video assisted thoracoscopic surgery

Fig. 1. Lymph node map and the modalities commonly used to biopsy lymph nodes.

INDICATIONS

The indications for mediastinal lymph node dissection include any disease process in which the pathologic evaluation of the nodal tissue affects treatment decisions. This occurs most often in patients with thoracic malignancy. Probably the most common indication for mediastinal lymph node dissection is during resection of a non–small cell lung cancer. The issue of complete resection of the mediastinal lymph nodes versus systematic sampling is somewhat controversial. Despite a recent randomized trial suggesting the adequacy of lymph node sampling, many surgeons (including the authors of this article) favor complete resection of the mediastinal nodes, provided it can be performed with minimal additional morbidity.[2] This is because the randomized study cited previously only studied patients who were lymph node negative on frozen section for stations 4R, 7, and 10R on the right and for stations 5, 7, and 10L on the left. The importance of pathologic evaluation of the mediastinal nodes in treating lung cancer relates to accurate staging, which further guides any potential adjuvant treatment. The same concept is applicable to other thoracic malignancies including esophageal cancer. Although a complete mediastinal lymph node dissection may not always be a component of pulmonary metastasectomy, lung metastases can also spread to the mediastinal lymph nodes, and the prognostic information gained from this pathologic assessment remains valuable.[3]

THORACOSCOPIC LYMPH NODE DISSECTION

Dissection of the mediastinal lymph nodes can be performed via thoracoscopic techniques and is typically a component of thoracoscopic lobectomies. Perhaps the most difficult aspect of video-assisted thoracic surgery (VATS) lobectomy is the lymph node dissection. There is no single standard port placement for thoracoscopic procedures, and techniques have been described using from 1 to 3 ports in addition to the utility incision.[4,5] The techniques for dissection include sharp dissection with scissors, use of electrocautery, and blunt dissection. For procedures in the right chest, the paratracheal space is opened by retracting the lung inferiorly. Following an upper lobectomy of the right lung, this space is easily accessed. The mediastinal pleura is divided superior to the azygos vein. If additional exposure is needed, the azygos vein can even be divided. The fatty tissue between the superior vena cava anteriorly and the trachea posteriorly is removed for a complete lymph node resection. Individual nodes can be identified and removed from this tissue for a lymph node sampling. Care must be taken not to injure the commonly seen small posterior venous branch that empties into the superior vena cava from the 4R or the small arterial branch that courses just medial to the trachea and goes to the 2R. The vagus nerve can also be injured as it crosses the trachea from the anterior side to the posterior side to its eventual position adjacent to the esophagus. Larger lymphatics

should be clipped or tied to minimize the risk of postoperative chylothorax.

The subcarinal space is accessed best from the right chest by retracting the lung medially. The mediastinal pleura is opened and the esophagus and vagus nerve are identified. The dissection is best started by hugging the pericardium and going up toward the right main stem bronchus. The connective tissue between the right and left main stem bronchi is dissected from the pericardium for a complete lymph node resection, or individual nodal fragments are removed for lymph node sampling. One disadvantage of lymph node sampling in this region is the bleeding that can be encountered from the raw surface of the lymph node. It is best to work around the node rather than inside it. Bleeding is often best controlled by removing the remainder of the nodal tissue while taking care to carefully control bronchial arterial branches within this area. There are typically 2 bronchial arterial branches that supply this nodal region: one that comes from the carina, which should be clipped, and the other that is smaller and comes from the esophagus near the vagus nerve branches. As described earlier, larger lymphatics that are identified should be controlled with clips to minimize the risk of postoperative chylothorax. To complete the lymph node dissection on the right side, the inferior pulmonary ligament is divided. The paraesophageal nodes are separated from the adjacent esophagus with preservation of the vagus nerve. Maintaining dissection medial to the vagus nerve allows complete nodal resection while minimizing the risk of injury to the nerve. After division of the inferior pulmonary ligament, the level 9 nodes are present in the connective tissue inferior to the inferior pulmonary vein. At the completion of the dissection, each of the operative sites should be examined for hemostasis, especially in the subcarinal and paratracheal spaces. If bleeding is present, this can often be controlled with cautery, direct pressure, or Surgicel (Ethicon, Somerville, NJ, USA). Bleeding from a bronchial artery requires direct control of the offending vessel.

A thoracoscopic lymph node dissection from the left chest includes opening the mediastinal pleura at the hilum to identify the superior pulmonary vein and left main pulmonary artery. The phrenic nerve anteriorly is preserved, and unipolar cautery should be limited in the aortopulmonary window to minimize the risk of injury to the recurrent laryngeal nerve. The nodes in levels 5 and 6 are removed. The subcarinal space, similar to the right side, is accessed by retracting the lung medially. Unlike the right side, however, the subcarinal space can be more difficult to access from the left side because of the aortic arch. Increasing the tidal volume to the right lung can help elevate the mediastinum to improve exposure. This level is much easier to assess robotically than with VATS. The third robotic arm should be used to retract the left upper lobe medially and cephalad to bring up the left main stem bronchus. Otherwise, the technical points outlined earlier for the right side are also applicable to the left side. As with the right side, the level 8 and 9 lymph nodes are completed after division of the inferior pulmonary ligament.

ROBOTIC DISSECTION OF MEDIASTINAL NODES

There has been a rapid increase in the use of the robot in thoracic surgery in the past year. It is now routinely being used for mediastinal, esophageal, and pulmonary procedures.[6] As a component of a pulmonary resection for malignancy, the robot provides a minimally invasive tool for complete thoracic lymph node removal. The technique of a completely portal robotic lobectomy with 4 arms has been previously described and championed at the authors' institution.[7] This specific port placement provides excellent exposure for the completion of mediastinal lymph node dissection. The authors and others have found it easier to perform a complete thoracic lymphadenectomy via the robot than via VATS, and have shown the efficacy of lymph node dissection.[4] Although the access to each lymph node region is similar to that described for thoracoscopy, the robotic approach offers several advantages.[8,9] The stereoscopic three-dimensional view with enhanced magnification provides precise anatomic detail. The degrees of movement of the robotic instrumentation allow more precise dissection in small spaces, such as the paratracheal and subcarinal spaces. The insufflation of carbon dioxide provides enough compression of the lung parenchyma and depression of the diaphragm to allow more working space within the hemithorax. As more surgeons incorporate the use of the robot in their pulmonary practice, the benefits it offers for the ease of lymph node dissection are often cited as one of the biggest advantages of robotics over VATS.

SUMMARY

The dissection of mediastinal (N2) lymph nodes is an integral part of the diagnosis, staging, and subsequent treatment of thoracic malignancies. A detailed understanding of the anatomy of these regions is paramount to performing a safe and efficient mediastinal lymph node dissection. The technology available today allows for a minimally invasive approach for lymph node sampling (endobronchial ultrasonography, esophageal ultrasonography) and for lymph node removal (VATS or robotic techniques). Although the use of robotics in thoracic surgery is relatively new, is expensive, and necessitates a learning curve for the entire team in the operating room, it offers several advantages in visualization and precision for lymph node dissection.

REFERENCES

1. Rusch VW, Asamura H, Watanabe H, et al. The IASLC lung cancer staging project: a proposal for a new international lymph node map in the forthcoming seventh edition of the TNM classification for lung cancer. J Thorac Oncol 2009;4:568–77.
2. Darling GE, Allen MS, Decker PA, et al. Randomized trial of mediastinal lymph node sampling versus complete lymphadenectomy during pulmonary resection in the patient with N0 or N1 (less than hilar) non-small cell carcinoma: results of the American College of Surgery Oncology Group Z0030 trial. J Thorac Cardiovasc Surg 2011;141:662–70.
3. Dominguez-Ventura A, Nichols FC. Lymphadenectomy in metastasectomy. Thorac Surg Clin 2006;16:139–43.
4. McKenna RJ Jr, Houck W, Fuller CB. Video-assisted thoracic surgery lobectomy: experience with 1,100 cases. Ann Thorac Surg 2006;81:421–6.
5. Onaitis MW, Petersen RP, Balderson SS, et al. Thoracoscopic lobectomy is safe and versatile procedure: experience with 500 consecutive patients. Ann Surg 2006;244:420–5.
6. Cerfolio RJ, Bryant AS, Minnich DJ. Starting a robotic program in general thoracic surgery: why, how, and lessons learned. Ann Thorac Surg 2011;91:1729–37.
7. Cerfolio RJ, Bryant AS, Skylizard L, et al. Initial consecutive experience of completely portal robotic pulmonary resection with 4 arms. J Thorac Cardiovasc Surg 2011;142:740–6.
8. Park BJ, Flores RM, Rusch VW. Robotic assistance for video-assisted thoracic surgical lobectomy: technique and initial results. J Thorac Cardiovasc Surg 2006;131:54–9.
9. Ninan M, Dylewski MR. Total port-access robot-assisted pulmonary lobectomy without utility of thoracotomy. Eur J Cardiothorac Surg 2010;38:231–2.

Video-Assisted Mediastinoscopic Lymphadenectomy and Transcervical Extended Mediastinal Lymphadenectomy

Marcin Zieliński, MD, PhD

KEYWORDS

- Lung cancer • Mediastinum • Surgery

Invasive staging of the mediastinal lymph nodes with the cervical mediastinoscopy is regarded as the gold standard of staging according to the current guidelines of the European Society of Thoracic Surgeons.[1] After the publication of the guidelines, however, the role of mediastinoscopy has been questioned by several investigators advocating the use of endoscopic techniques combined with ultrasonography, including endobronchial ultrasonography with transbronchial fine-needle biopsy (EBUS/TBNA) and endoesophageal ultrasonography and fine-needle aspiration (EUS).[2–4] The authors have reported that the diagnostic yield of EBUS and EUS was comparable or even better than that reported for standard mediastinoscopy. In the opinion of the authors, EBUS and EUS and, especially, EBUS/EUS combined might be preferred over mediastinoscopy because of the advantage of less invasiveness. During the last decade, however, 2 new invasive staging techniques representing more radical methods of mediastinal exploration have been introduced: video-assisted mediastinoscopic lymphadenectomy (VAMLA) and transcervical extended mediastinal lymphadenectomy (TEMLA).[5–10] These 2 techniques are intended for the complete removal of whole mediastinal nodes with the surrounding adipose tissue to improve the accuracy of staging instead of obtaining pieces of the nodes with the cervical mediastinoscopy introduced by Carlens in 1955.[11] The aim of this article is to compare VAMLA and TEMLA, the new procedures currently used by a limited number of thoracic surgeons.

MATERIAL AND METHODS

All publications and available meeting presentations were reviewed. Various parameters, such as the surgical technique, operative time, number of removed nodes and nodal stations, morbidity, mortality, diagnostic yield, use for repeated staging (restaging), and other important factors, were compared.

SURGICAL TECHNIQUE OF VAMLA

Preparation of the pretracheal space and introduction of the closed video mediastinoscope are the same as those used for standard mediastinoscopy.[5] By conventional preparation with the aspirator tube, first the bifurcation, both main bronchi and the left recurrent nerve are clearly identified.

On the left side, several lymph nodes become visible tracheobronchially next to the recurrent nerve. The optical enlargement in video mediastinoscopy and the bimanual preparation facilitate the removal of several complete left-sided lymph nodes despite the adjacent nerve.

When the subcarinal region is dissected, a specimen consisting of lymph nodes and the mediastinal fat tissue is first separated from the medial parts of both main bronchi and from the edge of

Department of Thoracic Surgery, Pulmonary Hospital, Ul Gładkie 1, 34 500 Zakopane, Poland
E-mail address: marcinz@mp.pl

Thorac Surg Clin 22 (2012) 219–225
doi:10.1016/j.thorsurg.2011.12.005
1547-4127/12/$ – see front matter © 2012 Elsevier Inc. All rights reserved.

Table 1
Comparison of surgical technique of VAMLA and TEMLA

Factor	VAMLA[5,7]	TEMLA[10]
Incision length	2–3 cm	5–8 cm
Method of removal of the nodes and the adipose tissue	2R, 4R, 2L, 4L, 7 Mediastinoscopy assisted	1, 2R, 4R, 2L, 4L, 7, 8, 3A, 3P, 5, 6 Classic open-fashion technique, stations 7, 8; 4L, mediastinoscopy assisted; stations 5 and 6, thoracoscopy assisted (through the cervical incision)
Mean operative time	54.1–74.0 min	128 min
Number of the removed nodes	8.6–20.7	37.9
Mortality	None	0.7% (30-d mortality unrelated causes)
Morbidity	4.0%	6.6%

the bifurcation. Then by distal dissection of about 3 cm, the complete subcarinal region is explored. The main bronchi can be exposed more easily on the right than on the left side ventrally toward the upper lobe origin. On the left side, the upper pulmonary vein becomes visible sometimes caudal to the pulmonary artery. Finally, the esophagus is exposed between the 2 main bronchi.

The right paratracheal and tracheobronchial compartments are mostly resected en bloc. Directly caudal to the innominate artery, the lymph nodes are grasped and pushed caudally to the left. Thus, the small cranial vascular and lymphatic attachments can be clearly dissected. Subsequently, the lymph nodes are drawn en bloc to the left and are dissected in a blunt fashion from the mediastinal pleura and the vena cava. Frequently, a clip has to be applied to a small venous branch originating from the vena cava. Now, at the right dorsal side of the trachea, the esophagus with the vagus nerve and after further caudal dissection, the junction of the azygos vein with the vena cava is exposed. As soon as the azygos vein is exposed, the lymph nodes are pulled in the left-cranial direction and are dissected from the distal margin of the tracheobronchial angle.

SURGICAL TECHNIQUE OF TEMLA

The operation starts with a 5- to 8-cm collar incision in the neck. The platysma muscle is divided and the anterior jugular veins are exposed, suture ligated, and divided. The visualization and protection of the laryngeal recurrent nerves bilaterally is a priority.[10]

After visualization of both laryngeal recurrent nerves, the sternal manubrium is elevated with a sharp 3-teeth hook connected to the Rochard frame (Aesculap Chifa, Nowy Tomysl, Poland) to widen the access to the mediastinum.

The highest mediastinal nodes (station 1 according to the Mountain-Dresler map) are dissected first.[12] These nodes are located above the upper margin of the left innominate vein and belong to the anterior lymphatic flow from the chest. The fatty tissue containing these nodes is dissected from the right carotid artery and the right innominate veins (laterally, on the right side), from the left carotid artery (laterally, on the left side), then it is dissected from the trachea (posteriorly) and from the left innominate vein (inferiorly). The piece of tissue containing the station 1 nodes is resected en block along with the upper poles of the thymus gland.

To enter the right paratracheal space containing stations 2R and 4R this is necessary to dissect along the right vagus nerve, which lies between the right carotid artery and the right jugular vein. The dissection proceeds along the nerve, below the division of the innominate artery. The origin of the right laryngeal recurrent nerve is clearly visible and protected from injury. The dissection proceeds toward the tracheal bifurcation. The whole fatty tissue containing the 2R and 4R nodes lying between the right innominate vein and the right mediastinal pleura (laterally), the ascending aorta and trachea (medially), the back wall of the superior vena cava (anteriorly) and the esophagus and the thoracic spine (posteriorly) and the right main bronchus, the azygos vein, and the right pulmonary artery (inferiorly) is removed.

The dissection of the left paratracheal nodes proceeds along the left laryngeal recurrent nerve below the level of the tracheal bifurcation. The nerve is dissected from the left wall of the trachea and the left main bronchus with a peanut sponge, whereas the lateral connections of the nerve are preserved to maintain the blood supply to the nerve. In most

Table 2
Differences in the extent of removal of the mediastinal nodes between VAMLA and TEMLA

	VAMLA[5,7]	TEMLA[10]
Incision	As for standard mediastinoscopy	5- to 8-cm collar incision in the neck; The platysma muscle is divided and the anterior jugular veins are exposed, suture-ligated, and divided
Visualization of the laryngeal recurrent nerve	Right nerve: not visualized Left nerve: identified at the level of the tracheal bifurcation and the left main bronchus	Both nerves visualized down from the level of the thyroid
Removal of the highest mediastinal nodes (station 1)	Not performed	Completely removed with the surrounding fatty tissue
Removal of 2R nodes	Performed in the mediastinoscopy-assisted technique	The open-fashion dissection of 2R proceeds in front of the innominate artery, along the right vagus nerve, below the division of the innominate artery; The origin of the right laryngeal recurrent nerve is clearly visible
Removal of 4R nodes	Completely removed with the surrounding fatty tissue in the mediastinoscopy-assisted technique	Completely removed with the surrounding fatty tissue in the open-fashion technique as a continuation of 2R removal
Removal of the prevascular (3A) and retro-tracheal (3P) stations	Not performed	Possible, performed optionally
Removal of the subcarinal nodes (station 7)	Completely removed with the surrounding fatty tissue in the mediastinoscopy-assisted technique	Completely removed with the surrounding fatty tissue in the mediastinoscopy-assisted technique
Removal of the periesophageal nodes (station 8)	Not mentioned	Completely removed within the reach of the Linder-Dahan mediastinoscope (19 cm)
Removal of the left upper paratracheal nodes (2L)	Removed if present (station inconsistently found)	Removed if present (station inconsistently found)
Removal of the left lower paratracheal nodes (4L)	Completely removed with visualization of the left laryngeal recurrent nerve	Completely removed with visualization of the left laryngeal recurrent nerve
Paraaortic, aorta-pulmonary window nodes (stations 5 and 6)	Not performed as a part of VAMLA but can be done as a part of the combined VAMLA/extended mediastinoscopy	Completely removed with the surrounding fatty tissue in the open-fashion technique

patients, the left upper paratracheal nodes (station 2L) are located medially and in front of the nerve, whereas the lower paratracheal nodes (station 4L) almost always lie behind the nerve. While carefully preserving the left laryngeal recurrent nerve, the lymph nodes, 2L and 4L, are dissected.

To enter the subcarinal nodes, it is necessary to divide the firm fascial layer covering the station 7 nodes anteriorly. The dissection proceeds along the medial walls of both main bronchi for the distance of 4 to 5 cm. The package containing the station 7 and 8 nodes is dissected from the

Table 3
Comparison of the diagnostic yield of VAMLA and TEMLA

	VAMLA[7]	TEMLA[13]
Number of patients	144	698
Sensitivity (%)	93.8	96.2
Specificity (%)	100	100
Negative predictive value (%)	Not stated	98.7
Positive predictive value (%)	Not stated	100
Accuracy (%)	Not stated	99.0

pulmonary artery and the pericardium covering the left atrium (anteriorly) and the esophagus (posteriorly) and removed en block.

For the removal of the subcarinal and periesophageal nodes (stations 7 and 8), the mediastinoscope is used; the author prefers the operative Linder-Dahan video mediastinoscope (Richard Wolf GmbH, Knittlingen, Germany) equipped with moving blades, which are very useful in retracting the pulmonary artery from the carina during the dissection of node station 7, and the left atrium from the esophagus during the dissection of node station 8, to a level 5 to 8 cm below the carina. The mediastinoscope is used for retracting these structures and visualization only; the removal of lymph nodes is performed using a standard dissector for open surgery, introduced through the right paratracheal space along the mediastinoscope. The Linder-Dahan mediastinoscope is also helpful in the removal of the most distal lower paratracheal nodes (station 4L). In these patients, the removal of the lower paratracheal nodes (station 4L) is postponed until the subcarinal and the periesophageal nodes are removed.

The entrance to the aorta-pulmonary window and station 6 nodes lies between the left innominate vein and the left carotid artery. The first step to reach this area is the division of the firm layer of the fascial tissue between the innominate artery, the left carotid artery, and the left innominate vein. The fascial layer obscures the view of these vessels and, after its division, the left innominate vein can be retracted anteriorly. After retracting the vein upwards using a long retractor, the plane is developed at the anterior surface of the aortic arch. With blunt dissection with a peanut sponge, the fatty tissue containing the station 6 nodes is dissected from the ascending aorta until the left pulmonary artery is reached. The left vagus nerve is a landmark of dissection. The nodes located above the convexity of the aortic arch and lying in front of the vagus nerve crossing the aortic arch and the Botallo ligament and the para-aortic nodes (station 6). The nodes located below the aortic arch and behind the Botallo ligament and the pulmonary-window nodes (station 5). The left pulmonary artery, the left phrenic nerve, and the left superior pulmonary vein are well visible after the completion of the dissection. If the mediastinal pleura opens, there is no need for the drainage of the mediastinum. The insertion of the piece of fibrin sponge and hyperinflation of the lungs during the closure of the wound is all that is necessary in such patients. The same rule is valid if the mediastinal pleura is opened on the right side.

Station 3A (prevascular nodes) and station 3P (retro-tracheal nodes) are removed in selected patients. Station 3A nodes lie below the left innominate vein, in front of the superior vena cava, medially to the right mediastinal pleura, and laterally to the ascending aorta. These nodes are dissected after the removal of station1 nodes. The left innominate vein and the superior vena cava are retracted

Table 4
Diagnostic sensitivity of the largest reported series of restaging of NSCLC

	De Waele et al[16] (Group 1) (Remediastinoscopy)	Marra et al[17] (Group 2) (Remediastinoscopy)	Herth et al[18] (Group 3) (EBUS)	Cerfolio et al[19] (Group 4) (PET/CT)	Zieliński et al[20] (Group 5) (TEMLA)
True positive	40	20	89	21	22
True negative	47	71	7	52	40
False positive	0	0	0	7	0
False negative	17	13	28	13	1
Overall	104	104	124	93	63

Comparison of sensitivity: groups 1–5 $P = .0156$; groups 2–5 $P = .0043$; groups 3–5 $P = .0357$; groups 4–5 $P = .0051$.

Comparison of negative predictive value: groups 1–5 $P = .0018$; groups 2–5 $P = .0312$; groups 3–5 $P = .0000$; groups 4–5 $P = .0105$.

Data from Zieliński M, Hauer L, Hauer J, et al. Non–small-cell lung cancer restaging with transcervical extended mediastinal lymphadenectomy. Eur J Cardiothorac Surg 2010;37:776–80.

Table 5
Comparison of diagnostic yield of EBUS/EUS and TEMLA for primary staging of NSCLC

Diagnostic Parameter	Primary Staging EBUS/EUS 617 Patients (%)	Primary Staging TEMLA 375 Patients (%)	Difference (P)
Sensitivity	88.9	98.6	P = .0000
Specificity	98.7	100	P = .0305
Negative predictive value	84.1	99.7	P = .0000
Positive predictive value	99.1	100	P = .0722

Data from Zieliński M, Szlubowski A, Kołodziej M, et al. Comparison of diagnostic yield of endoscopic ultrasound staging of non-small cell lung cancer (NSCLC) performed with use of endobronchial ultrasound (EBUS) and/or endoesophageal ultrasound (EUS) with invasive staging of NSCLC performed with use of transcervical extended mediastinal lymphadenectomy (TEMLA). 14th World Conference on Lung Cancer. Amsterdam, July 3–7, 2011. p. [abstract O03.01].

posteriorly with a peanut sponge, and the fatty tissue containing the 3A nodes is dissected from the structures mentioned previously. In the author's experience, these nodes are rarely the site of metastasis, only in the case of right-sided tumors.

The retro-tracheal nodes (station 3P) are located behind the bifurcation of the trachea. This area is approached in the same fashion as the right paratracheal nodes. The tracheal bifurcation is retracted anteriorly, which enables the visualization of the nodes lying in front of the esophagus. The nodes are easily removed; however, the author has never found any metastatic nodes in this station, and most often there are no visible nodes in this location at all. During TEMLA, all mediastinal lymph nodal stations and the surrounding fatty tissue are removed, with the exception of the pulmonary ligament station 9 nodes. The rule of TEMLA is to perform the lymphadenectomy in an en block fashion at least in part, with the resection of the whole package of the lymphatic tissue without separation of the individual nodes. It is possible to remove all the nodes of station 1 in one piece (also containing the upper poles of the thymus). Afterward, stations 2R and 4R are removed in one piece,

the same as stations 7 and 8 and 5 and 6. The author removes the nodes of stations 2L and 4L separately because they almost never occur in one piece of tissue.

Generally, most of TEMLA is an open procedure, with the exception of the dissection of the subcarinal nodes (station 7), the periesophageal (station 8) nodes, and the left lower paratracheal (station 4L) nodes, which are dissected in the mediastinoscopy-assisted fashion with the aid of the Linder-Dahan 2-blade mediastinoscope. The para-aortic station 6 and aorta-pulmonary window station 5 nodes are sometimes dissected with the aid of a video thoracoscope introduced to the mediastinum through the operative wound.

RESULTS

The search of PUBMED revealed 10 publications on VAMLA and 18 publications on TEMLA. The differences between VAMLA and TEMLA are presented in **Table 1**. The differences in the extent of the removal of the mediastinal nodes between VAMLA and TEMLA are shown in **Table 2**. The comparison of the diagnostic yield for VAMLA and TEMLA is shown in **Table 3**.[13]

Table 6
Comparison of diagnostic yield of EBUS/EUS and TEMLA for restaging of NSCLC after neoadjuvant treatment

Diagnostic Parameter	Restaging EBUS/EUS 52 Patients (%)	Restaging TEMLA 89 Patients (%)	Difference (P)
Sensitivity	79.2	95.5	P = .0023
Specificity	100	100	P = 1.000
Negative predictive value	84.8	98.5	P = .0015
Positive predictive value	100	100	P = 1.000

Abbreviation: NSCLC, non–small cell lung carcinoma.
Data from Zieliński M, Szlubowski A, Kołodziej M, et al. Comparison of diagnostic yield of endoscopic ultrasound staging of non-small cell lung cancer (NSCLC) performed with use of endobronchial ultrasound (EBUS) and/or endoesophageal ultrasound (EUS) with invasive staging of NSCLC performed with use of transcervical extended mediastinal lymphadenectomy (TEMLA). 14th World Conference on Lung Cancer. Amsterdam, July 3–7, 2011. p. [abstract O03.01].

There were no publications comparing VAMLA with standard mediastinoscopy. One publication prospectively compared TEMLA with standard mediastinoscopy. Because of the significantly better results of TEMLA, the study was canceled before the planned number of patients was included.[14] There was a single mention of 9 patients who underwent VAMLA after neoadjuvant chemotherapy or chemoradiotherapy.[7] No details about the use of VAMLA for restaging have been reported. The results on the use of and TEMLA in restaging compared with the results of the other restaging modalities (remediastinoscopy, EBUS, positron emission tomography [PET]/computed tomography [CT]) are presented in **Table 4**.[15–19]

There were no reports of the comparison of VAMLA and EBUS and EUS. The results of the comparison of TEMLA with EBUS and EUS are shown in **Tables 5** and **6**. The diagnostic yield of TEMLA was proved to be significantly better in comparison with EBUS and EUS for primary staging and for restaging (see **Tables 5** and **6**).[20]

VAMLA was successfully combined with video-assisted thoracic surgery (VATS) lobectomy, which improved the accuracy of intraoperative staging.[21] There was only a preliminary report of the combination of TEMLA with transcervical lobectomy, with no reports on the combination of TEMLA with the standard VATS lobectomy.[22] TEMLA was used as a part of the staging protocol for malignant mesothelioma.[23]

DISCUSSION

Both VAMLA and TEMLA represent the improved versions of mediastinoscopy and were described as "supermediastinoscopies."[24] The main advantage of both techniques in comparison with the standard mediastinoscopy is the possibility to remove the whole nodes with the surrounding fatty tissue instead of biopsies from the nodes as is taken during a mediastinoscopy. Because of this advantage, the diagnostic yields of VAMLA and TEMLA were much higher in comparison with the standard mediastinoscopy (as was proved for TEMLA).[14] Both techniques became feasible after the introduction of the 2-blade Linder-Dahan mediastinoscope, which enabled much wider access to the mediastinum; however, contrary to the VAMLA, most of the TEMLA procedure is performed in the open technique, without the use of a mediastinoscope. The nodal stations 1, 3A, 3P, 5, and 6 are not removed with VAMLA but can be removed by TEMLA. In the case of VAMLA, however, stations 5 and 6 can be reached with the use of additional extended mediastinoscopy. The other differences between VAMLA and

TEMLA include more nodal stations and the mean number of nodes removed with TEMLA in comparison with VAMLA (11 vs 5 nodal stations and 20.8 vs 37.9 nodes, respectively) but also shorter mean operative time (54 minutes for VAMLA vs 128 minutes for TEMLA) and lesser invasiveness of VAMLA. There was no mortality and lower morbidity after VAMLA and 0.3% mortality and 6.6% morbidity for TEMLA, it was not clear, however, if the results of VAMLA represented 30-day mortality and morbidity as was reported for TEMLA (the mortality of TEMLA was all caused by nonsurgical reasons). The diagnostic yield was slightly better for TEMLA than for VAMLA. It was not clear, however, if the results for VAMLA were calculated for all nodal stations or only for those accessible for VAMLA. The other difference between VAMLA and TEMLA was the elevation of the sternum with a special retractor connected with the Rochard frame, which widened the approach to the mediastinum and facilitated the performance of TEMLA. Such a maneuver has not been reported for VAMLA. TEMLA was used successfully for the staging of malignant mesothelioma and for the restaging of the mediastinal nodes after the neoadjuvant treatment of non–small cell lung carcinoma and proved to have a significantly better diagnostic yield than PET/CT, EBUS, EUS, and remediastinoscopy. There have been no reports on the use of VAMLA for staging or restaging of malignant mesothelioma.

The combination of a very extensive but still minimally invasive bilateral lymphadenectomy done by VAMLA or TEMLA with the other minimally invasive procedure (VATS lobectomy) has the advantage of accurate staging, possible therapeutic effect caused by bilateral lymphadenectomy, and possibly the preservation of the acceptable invasiveness of the whole combined operation.

REFERENCES

1. De Leyn P, Lardinois D, Van Schil PE, et al. ESTS guidelines for preoperative lymph node staging for non-small cell lung cancer. Eur J Cardiothorac Surg 2007;32:1–8.
2. Herth FJ, Krasnik M, Kahn N, et al. Combined endoscopic-endobronchial ultrasound-guided fine-needle aspiration of mediastinal lymph nodes through a single bronchoscope in 150 patients with suspected lung cancer. Chest 2010;138:790–4.
3. Vilmann P, Puri R. The complete 'medical' mediastinoscopy (EUS-FNA + EBUS-TBNA). Minerva Med 2007;98:331–8.
4. Annema JT, van Meerbeeck JP, Rintoul RC, et al. Mediastinoscopy vs endosonography for mediastinal

nodal staging of lung cancer: a randomized trial. JAMA 2010;304:2245–52.

5. Hurtgen M, Friedel G, Toomes H, et al. Radical video-assisted mediastinoscopic lymphadenectomy (VAMLA) – technique and first results. Eur J Cardiothorac Surg 2002;21:348–51.

6. Leschber G, Holinka G, Linder A. vid mediastinoscopic lymphadenectomy (VAMLA)–a method for systematic mediastinal lymph node dissection. Eur J Cardiothorac Surg 2003;24:192–5.

7. Witte B, Wolf M, Huertgen M, et al. Video-assisted mediastinoscopic surgery: clinical feasibility and accuracy of mediastinal lymph node staging. Ann Thorac Surg 2006;82:1821–7.

8. Kuzdzal J, Zielinski M, Papla B, et al. Transcervical extended mediastinal lymphadenectomy–the new operative technique and early results in lung cancer staging. Eur J Cardiothorac Surg 2005;27:384.

9. Zieliński M. Transcervical extended mediastinal lymphadenectomy: results of staging in two hundred fifty-six patients with non-small cell lung cancer. J Thorac Oncol 2007;2:370–2.

10. Zielinski M, Kuzdzal J, Nabialek T, et al. Transcervical extended mediastinal lymphadenectomy. Multimed Man Cardiothorac Surg 2006. DOI:10.1510/mmcts.2005.001693.

11. Carlens E. Mediastinoscopy. A method for inspection and tissue biopsy in the superior mediastinum. Chest 1959;36:343–52.

12. Mountain CF, Dresler CM. Regional lymph node classification for lung cancer staging. Chest 1997;111:1718.

13. Zielinski M, Hauer L, Hauer J, et al. Transcervical extended mediastinal lymphadenectomy (TEMLA) for staging and restaging of non-small-cell lung cancer (NSCLC). Pneumonol Alergol Pol 2011;79:196–206.

14. Kuzdzal J, Zielinski M, Papla B, et al. The transcervical extended mediastinal lymphadenectomy (TEMLA) versus cervical mediastinoscopy in NSCLC staging. Eur J Cardiothorac Surg 2007;31:88–94.

15. Zieliński M, Hauer L, Hauer J, et al. Non-small-cell lung cancer restaging with transcervical extended mediastinal lymphadenectomy. Eur J Cardiothorac Surg 2010;37:776–80.

16. De Waele M, Serra-Mitjans M, Hendriks J, et al. Accuracy and survival of repeat mediastinoscopy after induction therapy for non-small cell lung cancer in a combined series of 104 patients. Eur J Cardiothorac Surg 2008;33:824–8.

17. Marra A, Hillejan L, Fechner S, et al. Remediastinoscopy in restaging of lung cancer after induction therapy. J Thorac Cardiovasc Surg 2008;135:843–9.

18. Herth FJ, Annema JT, Eberhardt R, et al. Endobronchial ultrasound with transbronchial needle aspiration for restaging the mediastinum in lung cancer. J Clin Oncol 2008;26:3346–50.

19. Cerfolio RJ, Bryant AS, Ojha B. Restaging patients with N2 (stage IIIa) non-small cell lung cancer after neoadjuvant chemoradiotherapy: a prospective study. J Thorac Cardiovasc Surg 2006;131:1229–35.

20. Zieliński M, Szlubowski A, Kołodziej M, et al. Comparison of diagnostic yield of endoscopic ultrasound staging of non-small cell lung cancer (NSCLC) performed with use of endobronchial ultrasound (EBUS) and/or endoesophageal ultrasound (EUS) with invasive staging of NSCLC performed with use of transcervical extended mediastinal lymphadenectomy (TEMLA). 14th World Conference on Lung Cancer. Amsterdam, July 3–7, 2011. p. [abstract O03.01].

21. Witte B, Messerschmitt A, Hillebrand H, et al. Combined videothoracoscopic and videomediastinoscopic approach improves radicality of minimally invasive mediastinal lymphadenectomy for early stage lung carcinoma. Eur J Cardiothorac Surg 2009;35:343–7.

22. Zielinski M, Pankowski J, Hauer L, et al. The right upper lobe pulmonary resection performed through the transcervical approach. Eur J Cardiothorac Surg 2007;32:766–9.

23. Zielinski M, Hauer J, Hauer L, et al. Staging algorithm for diffuse malignant pleural mesothelioma. Interact Cardiovasc Thorac Surg 2010;10:185–9.

24. Rami-Porta R. Supermediastinoscopies: a step forward in lung cancer staging. J Thorac Oncol 2007;4:355–6.

The Role of Lymphadenectomy in Lung Cancer Surgery

Antonio D'Andrilli, MD[a],*, Federico Venuta, MD[b,c], Erino A. Rendina, MD[a]

KEYWORDS

- Lung cancer • Surgical treatment • Lymphadenectomy

The spread through the intrapulmonary, hilar, and mediastinal lymph nodes is a crucial pathway of diffusion for non–small cell lung cancer (NSCLC). The extent of lymph node involvement is the most significant factor influencing prognosis and therapeutic strategies.[1,2] Hence, adequate lymphadenectomy represents a fundamental procedure in lung cancer surgery for the achievement of accurate staging and potential survival benefit.

In current surgical practice, the options for intraoperative mediastinal lymph node assessment range from a simple palpatory inspection of the mediastinum to an extended bilateral lymph node dissection.

The surgeon's inability in determining the lymph node involvement without biopsy has been demonstrated in prospective studies. Gaer and Goldstraw,[3] on comparing the results of visual and palpatory intraoperative evaluation of lymph nodes with those of pathologic examination, reported a sensitivity of 71% and a positive predictive value of 64% if the histologic analysis is not performed.

Although a large amount of data has been reported in the literature, there is still no consensus regarding the extent of lymph node removal and the impact of lymphadenectomy on long-term prognosis.

Increasing information over time has allowed a better knowledge of the anatomic basis of lymphatic drainage patterns of the lungs, leading to the development of more precise indications for the choice of the most appropriate technique for lymph node removal when performing radical surgery.

Evidence from the literature and technical aspects of lymph node dissection are reported and discussed in this article.

LYMPH NODE DRAINAGE PATTERNS

Interlobar lymph nodes are the site of greatest incidence of intraparenchymal lymphatic metastases. These lymph nodes drain into the hilar nodes and then to the mediastinum.[4]

In less frequent conditions an aberrant drainage pattern can be present, which bypasses the intrapulmonary and hilar lymph nodes and proceeds directly to the mediastinal nodes, thus resulting in skip metastases. Most studies in the literature have demonstrated a great anatomic variability of the lymphatic system of the lungs, which justifies the difficulty of achieving high accuracy in predicting patterns of lymphatic spread from lung cancer.[5]

However, data from anatomic, pathologic, and clinical studies indicate that mediastinal drainage tends to be lobe dependent, because the location of the primary tumor may help to identify the mediastinal lymph node stations that are more likely to

The authors have nothing to disclose.

[a] Department of Thoracic Surgery, Sant'Andrea Hospital, University LaSapienza, Via di Grottarossa 1035, 00189 Rome, Italy

[b] Department of Thoracic Surgery, Policlinico Umberto I, University LaSapienza, Viale del Policlinico 155, 00161 Rome, Italy

[c] Fondazione Lorillard Spencer-Cenci, University La Sapienza, Piazzale A. Moro, 5, Rome, Italy

* Corresponding author.

E-mail address: adandrilli@hotmail.com

Thorac Surg Clin 22 (2012) 227–237
doi:10.1016/j.thorsurg.2011.12.001

be involved in the case of N2 disease, especially when a single metastatic station is present.[4,6,7]

In 1952 Borrie[8] published an anatomic investigation performed on resected specimens that provided fundamental information concerning the patterns of lung cancer lymphatic dissemination. These observations have been subsequently confirmed by several other studies.[5–7]

Right upper lobe tumors commonly tend to metastasize to the lower paratracheal (station 4) and pretracheal (station 3) nodes when a single-station N2 disease is present.[4,6,7,9–11] Isolated metastases to stations of the lower mediastinum are usually rare from tumors in this location. Involvement of subcarinal (station 7) and lower mediastinal (stations 8,9) nodes tends to be higher in those series analyzing patients with multi-station mediastinal disease.[11] Watanabe and colleagues,[11] in a study including patients with multilevel mediastinal involvement, found a 36% incidence of metastases to the lymph nodes of station 7.

Kotoulas and colleagues,[6] in a retrospective review of 557 patients with NSCLC who underwent lung resection and lymph node dissection, found that centrally located tumors from all lobes showed a significantly increased tendency to metastasize to station 7 nodes if compared with peripheral lesions.

Subcarinal lymph nodes are more commonly involved in right, middle, and lower lobe malignancies,[4,10,12] especially when there is an involvement of a single-station mediastinal lymph node. In the study by Nohr-Oser,[12] including 749 surgically treated patients with stage I to IV NSCLC, the incidence of metastasis to the subcarinal nodes was 1% from tumors of the right upper lobe and 13% from tumors of the right lower lobe. The middle lobe tumors tend to metastasize most frequently to the lower paratracheal nodes,[4] whereas the lower lobe drains into the lower mediastinal stations (paraesophageal and inferior pulmonary ligament).[4,6,9]

However, surgical and lymphoscintigraphic studies[13] have shown that the superior segment tumors in the lower lobe have a higher incidence of upper mediastinal metastases (mainly to station 4) if compared with the basilar segment tumors, probably because of the existence of a more direct lymphatic pathway.

Left upper lobe tumors tend to drain principally toward the aortopulmonary window (station 5) and the para-aortic (station 6) lymph nodes, with the former being the first mediastinal station through which metastasis occurs.[9,14,15]

Despite the relatively constant pattern of drainage, left upper lobe malignancies can metastasize to the subcarinal nodes and even to the lower mediastinal nodes, with a higher incidence if compared with the right upper lobe.[10,11] This less frequent pathway may be caused by the different drainage pattern of the lingula[4] that drains to the subcarinal lymph nodes first, followed by the aortopulmonary window and the periaortic stations.[4]

The paratracheal nodes are less frequently involved in tumors of the left upper lobe if compared with malignancies of the right upper lobe.[14]

Tumors of the left lower lobe, similar to those of the right lower lobe, drain most frequently to the subcarinal lymph nodes,[4,9,11,14] which is seen in patients with single-station mediastinal disease, whereas in multistation disease the aortopulmonary window nodes are commonly involved as well.[10] The lower mediastinal nodes, including paraesophageal and inferior pulmonary ligament station, have been found to be the next most frequently involved mediastinal sites.[9]

The left lower lobe, more than any other lobe, is the lobe with the highest propensity to metastasize to the contralateral mediastinal nodes.[7]

Based on literature data, studies evaluating the lymphatic spread patterns in patients with lung cancer N2 disease report an incidence from 18% to 38%[6,16–20] of patients with mediastinal nodes involved without metastatic hilar nodes (skip metastases). Most skip metastases involve single lymph node stations, and only in a minority of cases do they present as a multistation disease.[18,20]

Anatomic studies in the last decades[21,22] have provided an explanation of the skipping metastatic spread, demonstrating the existence of lung lymphatic vessels that run directly to the mediastinal lymph nodes, bypassing the intrapulmonary and hilar stations.

CLASSIFICATION OF LYMPH NODE INVOLVEMENT

Cahan and colleagues,[23] in 1951, were the first to provide a detailed description of a thorough hilar and mediastinal lymphadenectomy as a part of the operation for lung cancer. However, until the early 1970s the presence of metastatic mediastinal lymph nodes in lung cancer was considered as a factor precluding long-term survival, and was classified as N2 disease independently from the involvement of ipsilateral or contralateral nodes.

In 1978, Naruke and colleagues[24] presented an original article that proved the curability of a considerable number of patients with lung cancer who also have mediastinal metastasis. Nineteen percent of patients in this series survived at 5 years after lung resection and removal of the hilar and ipsilateral mediastinal lymph nodes. The location of the lymph nodes was reported according to a map of 14 lymph node stations for which anatomic definitions were used for the first time.

In 1983, the American Thoracic Society (ATS) underlined the lack of specificity in the definition of some lymph node stations in the Naruke map, and proposed a new system of clinical staging defining the node levels based on constant anatomic landmarks.[25]

In 1986, a Revised International Staging System was proposed by the American Joint Committee on Cancer and the Union Internationale Contre le Cancer.[26] This system maintained the 1983 ATS mapping, but created a distinction between the ipsilateral mediastinal lymph nodes with a better outcome, which were defined as N2, and the contralateral mediastinal nodes, which were classified together with the supraclavicular and the opposite hilar nodes as N3 disease, because of the significantly poorer prognosis.

In the subsequent Revision of Staging System published by Mountain in 1997,[27] only minor modifications were applied to the previous ATS pulmonary and mediastinal lymph node map. These modifications included the classification of nodes along the anterior surface of the main stem bronchus within the pleural reflection line as station 4 and N2 disease, and the classification of nodes in the midline of the mediastinum as N2 rather than N3. In the more recent editions of the lung cancer stage classification system, published in 2002[28] and 2009,[29] respectively, no significant changes were made in the N descriptors. Improved accuracy of the staging system over time has helped investigators to better define the role of lymph node dissection in lung cancer surgery. Development of a more precise universally accepted classification has proved fundamental in obtaining a rigorous definition of the level of involved lymph nodes and an appropriate assignation of each involved nodal level to the correct N stage.

TECHNIQUES FOR INTRAOPERATIVE LYMPH NODE REMOVAL AND EXTENT OF LYMPH NODE DISSECTION

There is general agreement on the principle that precise evaluation of the lymph node status is fundamental in lung cancer surgery to estimate prognosis, to give indications for oncologic therapy, and to compare results from different institutions. However, various techniques are used in current surgical practice for the intraoperative lymph node assessment and removal

associated with pulmonary resection, without definitive indications concerning the preferable option.

Furthermore, there is still no complete consensus on the terms used to define these techniques,[30] and this may produce a systematic bias when comparing the results from different studies.

In 2006 the European Society of Thoracic Surgeons[31] recommended definitions to describe intraoperative lymph node assessment modalities, including all available approaches from simple bioptic procedures to extended nodal dissection.

Selected lymph node biopsy is defined as the simple bioptic procedure of 1 or more suspicious lymph node stations, and is therefore justified only when resection is not feasible to prove the existence of N1 or N2 disease at exploratory thoracotomy.

By contrast, lymph node sampling (LNS) is the removal of 1 or multiple lymph nodes based on the preoperative or intraoperative findings that indicate a suspicion of metastatic involvement. Systematic sampling is performed based on a predetermined selection of lymph node stations specified by the surgeon.

Systematic nodal dissection (SND) is defined as the systematic removal of all the mediastinal tissue containing lymph nodes within anatomic landmarks, in association with intrapulmonary and hilar nodes. On the right side, in the upper mediastinal district it requires the removal of lymphatic tissue from an area bounded caudally by the take-off of the right upper lobe, superiorly by the innominate artery, anteriorly by the superior vena cava (SVC), and posteriorly by the trachea. Lymph nodes adjacent to the SVC and retrotracheal nodes should also be removed.

On the left side, at the level of the superior mediastinum, nodal dissection includes the lymphatic tissue in the area between the phrenic nerve anteriorly, the vagus nerve posteriorly, up to the top of the aortic arch superiorly, and caudally to the left main stem bronchus. Independently from the tumor side, complete removal of subcarinal nodes (all lymphatic tissue caudally to the carina and both main stem bronchi), the inferior pulmonary ligament nodes, and nodes adjacent to the caudal part of the esophagus should be accomplished. At the end of dissection the main stem bronchi, posterior pericardium, and esophagus should be completely free of lymphatic tissue.

SND on the left side, as proposed by Japanese investigators,[13,32,33] includes division of the ligamentum arteriosum and mobilization of the aortic arch, permitting a more extended removal of lymph nodes of stations from 2 to 4.

At present, the International Association for the Study of Lung Cancer recommends that at least 6 lymph node stations should be removed or sampled before the confirmation of N0 status. Three of these nodes/stations should be mediastinal, always including subcarinal, and 3 should be hilar.[34]

Lobe-specific systematic node dissection is defined as the excision of mediastinal tissue containing specific lymph node stations depending on the lobar location of the primary tumor, based on the anatomic analysis of specific lymphatic drainage patterns. This modality is generally accepted for selected clinical situations, such as the presence of peripheral squamous cell T1 carcinoma. In patients with such tumor characteristics undergoing a selective nodal dissection, the probability of unforeseen N2 disease is very low (<5%).[35]

The Bronchogenic Carcinoma Cooperative Group of the Spanish Society of Pneumology and Thoracic Surgery has recommended a minimal dissection of at least 3 mediastinal stations defined according to the lobar location of the tumor.[36] After removal and intraoperative histologic examination of the interlobar and hilar nodes, confirming the absence of N1 disease at frozen section analysis, the proposed lobe-specific mediastinal dissection includes the following node stations:

- Right upper and middle lobe: 2R, 4R, and 7
- Right lower lobe: 4R, 7, 8, and 9
- Left upper lobe: 5, 6, and 7
- Left lower lobe: 7, 8, and 9.

According to this lymphadenectomy proposal, the lymphatic specimen should include at least 6 nodes.

The most aggressive modality of lymphadenectomy described in the literature is the extended lymph node dissection, which is defined as the removal of bilateral, mediastinal, and cervical nodes through median sternotomy and cervicotomy. This approach has been proposed by Japanese surgeons,[13,37,38] mainly for the treatment of advanced-stage tumors and non–squamous cell histology tumors. The same procedure has been also used in other selected experiences of surgery for patients with initial diagnosis of N3 disease, after response to induction therapy.[39] Although these extended dissections allow for a thorough exploration of the mediastinum, such procedures have never gained wide acceptance because of their significant invasiveness.

Biopsy of the sentinel lymph node, which is currently used in the surgical treatment of other tumors such as breast cancer and melanoma, has been proposed more recently as a selective method to direct mediastinal lymph node dissection (MLND) in lung cancer. Results of some studies[40–42] have suggested that patients without disease in the hilar and mediastinal sentinel nodes may not require a mediastinal SND. However, the efficacy of this procedure is yet to be proved in randomized trials, and data regarding survival at long term are still limited.

In the current surgical practice, the SND and various modalities of mediastinal LNS, including partial or complete removal of selected nodal stations (with or without suspected metastases), have been reported to be the most used options.

Most investigators use the term mediastinal lymph node dissection when referring to SND. Moreover, when considering more selective procedures, the term LNS is frequently used to indicate both random sampling and systematic sampling. This lack of homogeneity in definitions has to be considered when comparing results from different studies.

Arguments supporting the use of MLND generally include improved radicality resulting from better local control and decreased risk of leaving undetected lymphatic micrometastases, which may determine a favorable impact on survival and staging.

Arguments against the routine use of MLND provided by proponents of mediastinal sampling include the increased risk for perioperative surgical morbidity, leading to prolonged hospitalization, and the lack of significant evidence for survival advantage. Moreover, an increase in operative time with MLND has been advocated as an additional element in favor of sampling procedures.

Different studies in the last decades have compared these 2 modalities (MLND and LNS) regarding their effect on long-term survival, recurrence rate, accuracy of pathologic staging, and surgical morbidity.

IMPACT OF LYMPHADENECTOMY ON SURVIVAL AND RECURRENCE RATE

A large amount of data has been published, mainly in the last 15 years, assessing the impact of lymph node dissection on prognosis and local tumor control in lung cancer surgery. Although the quality of the available scientific results is good, it is still not possible to achieve a definitive conclusion regarding the effect of the extent of lymph node removal on long-term survival and recurrence rate (**Tables 1** and **2**).

Table 1
Impact of lymph node dissection on survival: randomized studies

References	Stage	Patients		5-Year Survival (%)		
		MLND	LNS	MLND	LNS	*P* value
Sugi et al,[43] 1998	I (<2 cm)	59	56	81	84	N.S.
Izbicki et al,[44] 1998	I–IIIA	76	93	65.8	54.8	.25
Passlick et al,[45] 2002	I–IIIA	53	41	N.R.	N.R.	.27
Wu et al,[46] 2002	I–IIIA	268	264	82.1 (St. I)	57.4 (St. I)	.01
				50.4 (St. II)	34 (St. II)	.02
				26.9 (St. III)	6.1 (St. III)	.02
Darling et al,[47] 2011	T1–2, N0–1	525	498	67 (D.F.)	68 (D.F.)	.89

Abbreviations: D.F., disease free; N.R., not reported; N.S., not significant; St., stage.

A meta-analysis by Wright and colleagues[48] including 3 randomized controlled trials (RCTs)[43,44,46] was published in 2006, comparing survival results of patients undergoing lung resection for NSCLC associated with either MLND or LNS. In a pooled analysis, the chance of surviving longer than a 4-year period was higher in patients receiving MLND when compared with those receiving LNS, with an overall hazard ratio of 0.78.

Another previous meta-analysis by Menser and colleagues[15] on the same 3 randomized trials reported a reduced risk of death (pooled hazard ratio, 0.63) and a significantly lower recurrence rate in the MLND group.

However, if considering independently each RCT, different results can be observed and only the study by Wu and colleagues,[46] among those included in the aforementioned meta-analysis, showed a significant improvement in long-term prognosis for MLND over LNS at all tumor stages. The reported 5-year survival was 82% versus 57% at stage I (*P* = .01), 50% versus 34% at stage II (*P* = .02), and 27% versus 6% (*P* = .02) at stage III NSCLC following MLND and LNS, respectively.

When considering other trials assessing the impact of the extent of lymph node dissection on survival and recurrence rate, results may vary especially in relation to the stage of the disease.

In the largest RCT available in the literature, published by the American College of Surgeons Oncology Group (ACOSOG) in 2011,[47] 1111 patients with early-stage NSCLC have been enrolled by rigorous staging procedures (mediastinoscopy and intraoperative sampling of station 10) that allowed to confirm the N0 status at frozen-section analysis before lung resection. MLND or sampling was then performed according to a randomized assignation. Five-year disease-free survival was 67% for patients treated by MLND and 68% for those treated by LNS, without a significant difference between the 2 groups. Similarly, no significant difference was reported in terms of median survival (8.5 years in the MLND group and 8.1 years in the LNS group). Furthermore, there was no difference in local (*P* = .52), regional (*P* = .10), and distant (*P* = .76) recurrence rate between the 2 groups.

In another smaller randomized trial including 115 patients with NSCLC of less than 2 cm in diameter,

Table 2
Impact of lymph node dissection on recurrence rate: randomized studies

References	Stage	Patients		5-Year Survival (%)		
		MLND	LNS	MLND	LNS	*P* value
Izbicki et al,[44] 1998	I–IIIA	76	93	28.9 (local + distant)	31.2 (local + distant)	N.S.
Sugi et al,[43] 1998	I (<2 cm)	59	56	10 (local + distant)	13 (local + distant)	N.S.
Wu et al,[46] 2002	I–IIIA	240	231	2.9 (local)	4.8 (local)	N.R.
Darling et al,[47] 2011	T1–2, N0–1	525	498	5.7 (local)	4.8 (local)	.52
				5.9 (regional)	8.6 (regional)	.10

Abbreviations: N.R., not reported; N.S., not significant.

Sugi and colleagues[43] did not observe a significant difference in survival rate between patients undergoing MLND and patients undergoing LNS (81% vs 84% at 5 years). Also, the recurrence rate showed no significant difference between the 2 treatment groups.

These results observed in patients with early-stage NSCLC have been confirmed by several other nonrandomized studies.

Okada and colleagues,[49] in a large, controlled nonrandomized trial, reported a 5-year overall survival of 79% in the MLND group and 83% in the LNS group. According to multivariate analysis, the type of nodal dissection performed did not significantly affect either the disease-free survival ($P = .63$) or the overall survival ($P = .11$).

A retrospective analysis performed by Doddoli and colleagues[50] showed no significant difference at univariate analysis in 5-year survival between patients receiving MLND (64%) and patients receiving sampling (59%) for stage I NSCLC. However, MLND was found to be a significant favorable prognostic factor at multivariate analysis ($P = .048$).

Another interesting retrospective study has been conducted on 442 patients with stage I NSCLC by Gajra and colleagues,[51] who found a 5-year survival rate of 85.9% after MLND and of 83.3% after systematic sampling, with no significant difference between the 2 treatment options. By contrast, patients undergoing random sampling in this study reported a significantly worse prognosis (56.4% survival at 5 years).

Two prospective randomized studies[44,45] assessing the impact of lymph node dissection on long-term prognosis in patients with stage I to III tumors observed no overall survival advantage in patients treated by lung resection with SND.

However, in one of these trials Passlick and colleagues[45] noted a significant survival benefit related to MLND in the subgroup of patients without micrometastases on histochemical testing.

In the other study, published by Izbicki and colleagues,[44] overall survival was higher after MLND (65.8% at 5 years) than after LNS (54.8% at 5 years), but this difference was not statistically significant. Similarly, the recurrence rate did not show a significant difference between the 2 treatment arms, but MLND prolonged relapse-free survival ($P = .037$) in patients with N1 and single-station N2 disease.

In contrast to results of most studies in the literature, Lardinois and colleagues,[52] in a nonrandomized trial including 100 patients with clinical stage T1 to T3, N0 to N1 NSCLC, found a significant advantage in disease-free survival related to the use of SND only for patients with stage I NSCLC (median [standard deviation]: 60.2 [7] months with MLND vs 44.8 [8] months with LNS; $P<.03$), but there was no significant difference between the 2 treatment options when considering patients at all stages. Also, the local recurrence rate was found to be lower in the MLND group only in patients with stage I NSCLC (12.5% vs 45%; $P = .02$) and in patients with negative mediastinum at pathologic staging (13% vs 46%; $P = .004$). However, the significance of the results reported in the latter study may be limited by the small statistical sample and by a possible bias in the inclusion criteria, because the assignation of patients to each treatment modality was based on personal choice of the surgeons, as pointed out by the investigators.

Different results can be found in those studies assessing the role of lymph node dissection in patients with advanced-stage NSCLC.

Zhang and colleagues[53] reported a median survival of 23.5 months in patients undergoing MLND and of 20 months in patients undergoing LNS for stage III NSCLC ($P<.05$). MLND was also a favorable predictor of survival at multivariate analysis.

Keller and colleagues[54] enrolled patients with stage II and stage IIIA NSCLC in a comparative nonrandomized study. The median survival was 57.5 months for the 186 patients who had undergone MLND and 29.2 months for the 187 patients who had undergone LNS, with a statistically significant difference ($P = .004$) between the 2 groups.

ACCURACY OF STAGING

Accuracy in the definition of tumor stage represents a crucial issue in lung cancer surgery. Incomplete removal of lymphatic tissue when metastatic involvement is present may negatively influence postoperative treatment strategy by avoiding adjuvant therapy administration, and may compromise the validity of oncologic results by underestimating the tumor extension.

In the last years, several studies have been conducted with the aim of assessing the impact of the extent of lymph node dissection on the accuracy of staging. The resulting data provide some conflicting indications.

Keller and colleagues,[54] in a nonrandomized analysis, found N1 disease in 41% of the 186 patients treated by complete mediastinal dissection compared with 40% of the 187 patients receiving sampling ($P = .92$). Also, the reported N2 disease rate was similar between the 2 groups (20% in the MLND patients and 21% in the LNS patients). However, among patients with mediastinal node metastases, multiple N2 levels were documented in 30% of patients receiving MLND and in 12% of patients treated by LNS. This difference was statistically significant (P = .001), suggesting the possibility of a better definition of the mediastinal extension of the disease by a complete removal of the lymphatic tissue.

Similar results have been previously reported from a randomized trial by Izbicki and colleagues.[55] No significant difference was observed in tumor staging between the MLND group and the LNS group. However, as in the Keller study, the rate of patients with N2 disease presenting multilevel involvement was found to be significantly higher after MLND (57.2%) than after LNS (17.4%; P = .007). The number of patients with skip metastases was higher after sampling (30.4%) than after systematic lymphadenectomy (18.2%).

Other studies have provided different indications concerning the impact of lymph node dissection on tumor staging, showing significantly higher rates of patients with N2 disease after MLND. Wu and colleagues,[46] in a randomized trial including 532 patients, found a 48% stage III rate in the MLND group and a 28% stage III rate in the mediastinal sampling group. In the sampling group of this study, mediastinal lymph nodes were removed only if suspicious.

Massard and colleagues[56] performed a multicenter cross-sectional study including 208 patients with operable NSCLC. A mediastinal LNS was performed before resection to compare its pathologic results with those of the MLND performed subsequently. Mediastinal sampling was able to identify only 52% of cases with N2 disease and 40% of cases with multilevel N2 discovered by the SND.

Gajra and colleagues[51] classified the 442 patients at stage I included in their retrospective study into quartiles according to the number of nodes harvested: less than 4, 4 to 6, 7 to 9, and more than 9. The corresponding 5-year disease-free survival rates were 47.3%, 72.8%, 76.4%, and 79.1%, respectively. Five-year survival when 4 or more mediastinal nodal stations were removed was 87.6%. The investigators concluded that the higher number of lymph nodes and stations harvested significantly influenced the probability to achieve an accurate definition of stage I disease, which may have had a favorable impact on prognosis.

According to results from the randomized study by Sugi and colleagues,[43] the rate of unsuspected N2 disease found at definitive pathologic examination after MLND (12%) was not higher than that observed after LNS (14%).

In the ACOSOG Z0030 protocol,[47] which excluded patients with N2 disease, absence of mediastinal lymph nodes was confirmed before randomization by a mediastinoscopic, thoracotomic, or video-assisted thoracic surgery (VATS) systematic sampling. In addition, sampling of any suspicious node was performed. This process allowed elimination of most patients with N2 occult positive mediastinal nodes, thus justifying a lower incidence (4%) of unsuspected N2 disease at final pathologic examination.

COMPLICATIONS OF LYMPH NODE DISSECTION

One of the main arguments advocated by proponents of LNS against the choice of MLND is the potentially increased risk of complications associated with a more extended procedure. Possible related complications include bleeding; bronchial stump insufficiency caused by a more extended bronchial devascularization, resulting in fistula; laryngeal nerve palsy; impairment of lymphatic back flow with pulmonary edema; and respiratory distress syndrome.[57]

Several studies in the literature, including some randomized trials, have compared SND with LNS, assessing the risk of surgical morbidity related to these 2 procedures. In the largest prospective randomized trial conducted by the ACOSOG (Z0030),[58] no difference was observed in the incidence of complications (atrial arrhythmia, respiratory failure, chylothorax, persistent air leaks, recurrent nerve injury) between patients undergoing MLND and those undergoing sampling. Also, the duration of postoperative in-hospital stay and chest drain presented no difference between the 2 groups, although the time of operation was prolonged by a median of 14 minutes when MLND was performed.

Similarly, in the other large randomized trial by Wu and colleagues,[46] equal morbidity between patients undergoing systematic lymphadenectomy and patients receiving sampling was reported.

Izbicki and colleagues[59] performed an analysis of morbidity in a smaller randomized study. Also, in this trial the complication rate was not affected by the technique of lymph node removal used with lung resection. In particular, recurrent laryngeal nerve palsy was reported in 6 patients of the systematic sampling group and in 5 patients of SND group. One chylothorax occurred in each group. Although SND prolonged the operative time of about 20 minutes, there was no increase in blood loss, need for reoperation, and mortality. Also, duration of chest drain and length of hospitalization were similar in the 2 groups.

Keller and colleagues,[54] in a multicenter non-randomized study on 373 patients, showed that MLND does not entail increased blood loss and mean operative time when compared with sampling.

Doddoli and colleagues,[50] in a retrospective analysis, reported no difference in complication rate between the 2 techniques of nodal exeresis, except for the occurrence of laryngeal nerve palsy that was higher after systematic dissection.

In the smaller study by Lardinois and colleagues,[52] MLND required a significantly longer operation time than LNS ($P<.001$), but there was no significant difference between the 2 treatment options in terms of duration of chest-tube drainage (6.8 ± 4.2 vs 6.8 ± 4.3 days; $P = 1$), hospitalization (16.4 ± 5.4 vs 15.8 ± 6.6 days; $P = .62$), and morbidity. There was no recurrent nerve palsy, and phrenic nerve palsy was observed in one patient in each group.

Bollen and colleagues[60] have analyzed the postoperative complications of 155 patients with NSCLC who were treated by complete MLND (n = 65), systematic sampling (n = 20), or no MLND (n = 70). Intraoperative blood loss and the need for transfusion were not significantly different among the 3 treatment options. Bronchopleural fistula developed in 2 patients who had not undergone node dissection, while recurrent laryngeal nerve palsy was observed in 3 patients who underwent complete MLND.

SURGICAL APPROACHES FOR MLND

MLND is most frequently performed through a posterolateral or a lateral thoracotomy because most patients with NSCLC undergoing surgery are operated on through an open access.[61–63]

However, because of the recent progressive affirmation of VATS even in oncologic major lung resections,[64] the incidence of lymph node dissection procedures performed by a thoracoscopic approach is increasing over time.

Although several retrospective data can be found in the literature, only few small prospective trials have compared the VATS and thoracotomy approaches regarding MLND.

In the prospective randomized trial by Sugi and colleagues,[65] a total of 100 patients with clinical stage I NSCLC who were undergoing lobectomy by VATS (n = 50) or thoracotomy (n = 50) were included. Two of the patients in the VATS group required conversion to open surgery. The number of lymph nodes harvested was equal in the 2 groups, with a mean of 8 hilar and 13 mediastinal lymph nodes. The actuarial 5-year survival was similar: 90% after VATS and 85% after open

resection. Although a slightly higher locoregional recurrence rate (19%) was observed after thoracotomy in comparison with the VATS approach (10%).

Sagawa and colleagues[66] have published another prospective study including 35 patients with clinical stage I NSCLC who underwent VATS lobectomy with MLND. After the thoracoscopic procedure, a small thoracotomy was performed by a different surgeon to assess the completeness of the lymphadenectomy. Conversion to thoracotomy for the accomplishment of lobectomy was required in 6 patients. On the right side, a mean of 40.3 lymph nodes were removed by VATS, and a mean of 1.2 (range 0–6) additional lymph nodes were harvested by thoracotomy. On the left side, VATS allowed removal of a mean of 37.1 nodes while a mean of 1.2 additional nodes were resected by thoracotomy. The reported rate of lymph nodes missed by VATS (2%–3%) was considered acceptable for clinical stage I by the investigators.

More recently, Kuzdzal and colleagues[67] have described a new technique of transcervical extended mediastinal lymphadenectomy. The procedure is performed through a collar incision, with a videomediastinoscopy-assisted technique using a sternal elevating retractor, and allows dissection of lymph node stations 2R/L, 3a, 4R/L, 5, 6, 7, and 8. In a prospective study, thoracotomy has been performed in patients without mediastinal metastases, to accomplish lung resection and to search for any missed lymph node. The reported sensitivity, specificity, and accuracy of the transcervical procedure were high: 90%, 100%, and 96%, respectively.

ACKNOWLEDGMENTS

The authors wish to thank Dr Elisabetta Grigioni for data management and editorial revision.

REFERENCES

1. Rendina EA, Venuta F, De Giacomo T, et al. Stage IIIB non-small-cell lung cancer. Chest Surg Clin N Am 2001;11(1):101–19.
2. Rendina EA, Venuta F, De Giacomo T, et al. Induction chemotherapy for T4 centrally located non-small cell lung cancer. J Thorac Cardiovasc Surg 1999;117(2):225–33.
3. Gaer JA, Goldstraw P. Intraoperative assessment of nodal staging at thoracotomy for carcinoma of the bronchus. Eur J Cardiothorac Surg 1990;4:207.
4. Asamura H, Nakayama H, Kondo H, et al. Lobe-specific extent of systematic lymph node dissection for non-small cell lung carcinomas according to

a retrospective study of metastasis and prognosis. J Thorac Cardiovasc Surg 1999;117(6):1102–11.

5. Lardinois D, Brack T, Gaspert A, et al. Broncho-scopic radioisotope injection for sentinel lymph node mapping in potentially resectable non-small-cell lung cancer. Eur J Cardiothorac Surg 2003;23:824–7.

6. Kotoulas CS, Foroulis CN, Kostikas K, et al. Involve-ment of lymphatic metastatic spread in non-small cell lung cancer accordingly to the primary cancer location. Lung Cancer 2004;44(2):183–91.

7. Kim AW. Lymph node drainage patterns and micro-metastasis in lung cancer. Thorac Cardiovasc Surg 2009;21:298–308.

8. Borrie J. Primary carcinoma of the bronchus: prog-nosis following surgical resection. Ann R Coll Surg Engl 1952;10:165.

9. Turna A, Solak O, Kilicgun A, et al. Is lobe-specific lymph node dissection appropriate in lung cancer patients undergoing routine mediastinoscopy? Thor-ac Cardiovasc Surg 2007;55(2):112–9.

10. Ichinose Y, Kato H, Koike T, et al, Japanese Clinical Oncology Group. Completely resected stage IIIA non-small cell lung cancer: the significance of primary tumor location and N2 station. J Thorac Car-diovasc Surg 2001;122(4):803–8.

11. Watanabe Y, Shimizu J, Tsubota M, et al. Mediastinal spread of metastatic lymph nodes in bronchogenic carcinoma. Mediastinal nodal metastases in lung cancer. Chest 1990;97(5):1059–65.

12. Nohl-Oser HC. An investigation of the anatomy of the lymphatic drainage of the lungs as shown by the lymphatic spread of bronchial carcinoma. Ann R Coll Surg Engl 1972;51(3):157–76.

13. Hata E, Hayakawa K, Miyamoto H, et al. Rationale for extended lymphadenectomy for lung cancer. Theor Surg 1990;5:19.

14. Naruke T, Tsuchiya R, Kondo H, et al. Lymph node sampling in lung cancer: how should it be done? Eur J Cardiothorac Surg 1999;16(Suppl 1):S17–24.

15. Manser R, Wright G, Hart D, et al. Surgery for early stage non-small cell lung cancer. Cochrane Data-base Syst Rev 2005;1:CD004699.

16. Okada M, Sakamoto T, Yuki T, et al. Border between N1 and N2 stations in lung carcinoma: lessons from lymph node metastatic patterns of lower lobe tumors. J Thorac Cardiovasc Surg 2005;129(4):825–30.

17. Riquet M, Assouad J, Bagan P, et al. Skip medias-tinal lymph node metastasis and lung cancer: a particular N2 subgroup with a better prognosis. Ann Thorac Surg 2005;79(1):225–33.

18. Ilic N, Petricevic A, Arar D, et al. Skip mediastinal nodal metastases in the IIIa/N2 non-small cell lung cancer. J Thorac Oncol 2007;2(11):1018–21.

19. Liptay MJ, Grondin SC, Fry WA, et al. Intraoperative sentinel lymph node mapping in non-small-cell lung cancer improves detection of micrometastases. J Clin Oncol 2002;20(8):1984–8.

20. Prenzel KL, Mönig SP, Sinning JM, et al. Role of skip metastasis to mediastinal lymph nodes in non-small cell lung cancer. J Surg Oncol 2003;82(4):256–60.

21. Riquet M, Hidden G, Debesse B. Direct lymphatic drainage of lung segments to the mediastinal nodes. An anatomic study on 260 adults. J Thorac Cardio-vasc Surg 1989;97:623–32.

22. Riquet M. Anatomic basis of lymphatic spread from carcinoma of the lung to the mediastinum: surgical and prognostic implications. Surg Radiol Anat 1993;15:271–7.

23. Cahan WG, Watson WL, Pool JL. Radical pneumo-nectomy. J Thorac Surg 1951;22(5):449–73.

24. Naruke T, Suemasu K, Ishikawa S. Lymph node mapping and curability at various levels of metas-tasis in resected lung cancer. J Thorac Cardiovasc Surg 1978;76(6):832–9.

25. American Thoracic Society. Medical section of the American Lung Association. Clinical staging of primary lung cancer. Am Rev Respir Dis 1983;127(5):659–64.

26. Mountain CF. A new international staging system for lung cancer. Chest 1986;89(Suppl 4):225S–33S.

27. Mountain CF. Revisions in the international system for staging lung cancer. Chest 1997;111(6):1710–7.

28. Union Internationale Contre le Cancer. TNM classifi-cation of malignant tumors. 6th edition. New York: Wiley-Liss; 2002. p. 272.

29. Detterbeck FC, Boffa DJ, Tanoue LT. The new lung cancer staging system. Chest 2009;136(1):260–71.

30. Barnard J, Dunning J, Musleh G, et al. Is there a role for the use of radical lymph node dissection in the surgical management of resectable non-small cell lung cancer? Interact Cardiovasc Thorac Surg 2004;3(2):294–9.

31. Lardinois D, De Leyn P, Van Schil P, et al. ESTS guidelines for intraoperative lymph node staging in non-small cell lung cancer. Eur J Cardiothorac Surg 2006;30(5):787–92.

32. Watanabe Y, Shimizu J, Oda M, et al. Improved survival in left non-small-cell N2 lung cancer after more extensive operative procedure. Thorac Cardio-vasc Surg 1991;39:89.

33. Nakahara K, Fujii Y, Matsumura A, et al. Role of systematic mediastinal dissection in N2 non-small cell lung cancer patients. Ann Thorac Surg 1993;56:331.

34. Goldstraw P. International Association for the Study of Lung Cancer handbook in thoracic oncology. Orange Park (FL): Editorial Rx Press; 2009.

35. De Leyn P, Vansteenkiste J, Cuypers P, et al. Role of cervical mediastinoscopy in staging of non small cell lung cancer without enlarged mediastinal lymph no-des on CT-scan. Eur J Cardiothorac Surg 1997;12:706–12.

36. GCCB (Grupo Coperativo de Carcinoma Broncoge-nico de la Sociedad Espanola de Neumologia y Cirugia Toracica. Intraoperative lymph node staging in bronchogenic carcinoma. Consensus Report. Arch Bronconeumol 2001;37:495–503.

37. Hata E, Miyamoto H, Tanaka M, et al. Superradical operation for lung cancer: bilateral mediastinal dissection (BMD) with or without cervical dissection (CD). Lung Cancer 1994;11(Suppl 2):41.

38. Mitsuoka M, Hayashi A, Takamori S, et al. The signif-icance of lymph nodes (LN) dissection through median sternotomy for left lung cancer. Lung Cancer 1994;11(Suppl 1):149.

39. D'Andrilli A, Venuta F, Rendina EA. Resection for patients initially diagnosed with N3 after response to induction therapy. In: Ferguson MK, editor. Diffi-cult decisions in thoracic surgery: an evidence-based approach. New York: Springer; 2007. p. 128–39.

40. Melfi FM, Chella A, Menconi GF, et al. Intraoperative radioguided sentinel lymph node biopsy in non-small cell lung cancer. Eur J Cardiothorac Surg 2003;23:214.

41. Faries MB, Bleicher RJ, Ye X, et al. Lymphatic mapping and sentinel lymphadenectomy for primary and metastatic pulmonary malignant neoplasms. Arch Surg 2004;139:870.

42. Nomori H, Watanabe K, Ohtsuka T, et al. In vivo identification of sentinel lymph nodes for clinical stage I non-small cell lung cancer for abbreviation of mediastinal lymph node dissection. Lung Cancer 2004;46:49.

43. Sugi K, Nawata K, Fujita N, et al. Systematic lymph node dissection for clinically diagnosed peripheral non-small-cell lung cancer less than 2 cm in diameter. World J Surg 1998;22(3):290–4 [discussion: 294–5].

44. Izbicki JR, Passlick B, Pantel K, et al. Effectiveness of radical systematic mediastinal lymphadenectomy in patients with resectable non-small cell lung cancer: results of a prospective randomized trial. Ann Surg 1998;227(1):138–44.

45. Passlick B, Kubuschock B, Sienel W, et al. Medias-tinal lymphadenectomy in non-small cell lung cancer: effectiveness in patients with or without nodal micrometastases—results of a preliminary study. Eur J Cardiothorac Surg 2002;21(3):520–6.

46. Wu Y, Huang ZF, Wang SY, et al. A randomized trial of systematic nodal dissection in resectable non-small cell lung cancer. Lung Cancer 2002;36(1):1–6.

47. Darling GE, Allen MS, Decker PA, et al. Randomized trial of mediastinal lymph node sampling versus complete lymphadenectomy during pulmonary resection in the patient with N0 or N1 (less than hilar) non-small cell carcinoma: results of the American College of Surgery Oncology Group Z0030 Trial. J Thorac Cardiovasc Surg 2011;141(3):662–70.

48. Wright G, Manser RL, Byrnes G, et al. Surgery for non-small cell lung cancer: systematic review and meta-analysis of randomised controlled trials. Thorax 2006;61(7):597–603.

49. Okada M, Sakamoto T, Yuki T, et al. Selective medi-astinal lymphadenectomy for clinico-surgical stage I non-small cell lung cancer. Ann Thorac Surg 2006; 81(3):1028–32.

50. Doddoli C, Aragon A, Barlesi F, et al. Does the extent of lymph node dissection influence outcome in patients with stage I non-small-cell lung cancer? Eur J Cardiothorac Surg 2005;27(4):680–5.

51. Gajra A, Newman N, Gamble GP, et al. Effect of number of lymph nodes sampled on outcome in patients with stage I non-small-cell lung cancer. J Clin Oncol 2003;21(6):1029–34.

52. Lardinois D, Suter H, Hakki H, et al. Morbidity, survival, and site of recurrence after mediastinal lymph-node dissection versus systematic sampling after complete resection for non-small cell lung cancer. Ann Thorac Surg 2005;80(1):268–74 [discussion: 274–5].

53. Zhang GQ, Han F, Gao SL, et al. Two patterns of mediastinal lymph node resection for non-small cell lung cancer of stage IIIA: survival analysis of 219 cases. Ai Zheng 2007;26(5):519–23 [in Chinese].

54. Keller SM, Adak S, Wagner H, et al. Mediastinal lymph node dissection improves survival in patients with stages II and IIIa non-small cell lung cancer. Eastern Cooperative Oncology Group. Ann Thorac Surg 2000;70(2):358–65 [discussion: 365–6].

55. Izbicki JR, Passlick B, Karg O, et al. Impact of radical systematic mediastinal lymphadenectomy on tumor staging in lung cancer. Ann Thorac Surg 1995;59(1):209–14.

56. Massard G, Ducrocq X, Kochetkova EA, et al. Sampling or node dissection for intraoperative staging of lung cancer: a multicentric cross-sectional study. Eur J Cardiothorac Surg 2006; 30(1):164–7.

57. De Giacomo T, Venuta F, Rendina EA. Role of lym-phadenectomy in the treatment of clinical stage I non-small cell lung cancer. Thorac Surg Clin 2007; 17(2):217–21.

58. Allen MS, Darling G, Pechet T, et al. Morbidity and mortality of major pulmonary resections in patients with early stage lung cancer: initial results of the randomized, prospective ACOSOG Z0030 trial. Ann Thorac Surg 2006;81:1013–20.

59. Izbicki JR, Thetter O, Habekost M, et al. Radical systematic mediastinal lymphadenectomy in non-small cell lung cancer: a randomized controlled trial. Br J Surg 1994;81:229.

60. Bollen EC, van Duin CJ, Theunissen PH, et al. Medi-astinal lymph node dissection in resected lung

cancer: morbidity and accuracy of staging. Ann Thorac Surg 1993;55:961.

61. Rendina EA, Venuta F, De Giacomo T, et al. Safety and efficacy of bronchovascular reconstruction after induction chemotherapy for lung cancer. J Thorac Cardiovasc Surg 1997;114(5):830–5 [discussion: 835–7].

62. D'Andrilli A, Venuta F, Menna C, et al. Extensive resections: pancoast tumors, chest wall resections, en bloc vascular resections. Surg Oncol Clin N Am 2011;20:733–56.

63. Venuta F, Ciccone AM, Anile M, et al. Reconstruction of the pulmonary artery for lung cancer: long-term results. J Thorac Cardiovasc Surg 2009;138(5):185–91.

64. De Giacomo T, Rendina EA, Venuta F, et al. Thoracoscopic staging of IIIB non-small cell lung cancer before neoadjuvant therapy. Ann Thorac Surg 1997;64(5):1409–11.

65. Sugi K, Kaneda Y, Esato K. Video-assisted thoracoscopic lobectomy reduces cytokine production more than conventional open lobectomy. Jpn J Thorac Cardiovasc Surg 2000;48:161.

66. Sagawa M, Sato M, Sakurada A, et al. A prospective trial of systematic nodal dissection for lung cancer by video-assisted thoracic surgery: can it be perfect? Ann Thorac Surg 2002;73:900.

67. Kuzdzał J, Zieliński M, Papla B, et al. Transcervical extended mediastinal lymphadenectomy–the new operative technique and early results in lung cancer staging. Eur J Cardiothorac Surg 2005;27(3):384–90 [discussion: 390].

The Impact of Complete Lymph Node Dissection for Lung Cancer on the Postoperative Course

Hiroshi Date, MD

KEYWORDS

- Lung cancer • Lymph node dissection
- Lymph node sampling • Lymph node biopsy
- Survival • Staging

It is well known that metastasis to hilar or mediastinal lymph node, the N factor, is one of the most important determinants of prognosis after lung cancer surgery.[1–3] However, the role of lymphadenectomy in the staging and treatment of non–small cell lung cancer (NSCLC) remains controversial. Current surgical practice varies from visual inspection of the unopened mediastinum to systematic lymph node dissection (LND). Systematic mediastinal LND, as practiced by Japanese surgeons, is a much more extensive operation than that practiced by North American surgeons. Little and colleagues[4] surveyed 729 hospitals to retrieve information on the patterns of surgical care provided to patients with NSCLC. The report included more than 11,000 patients with major pulmonary resections and showed that only 57.3% of patients had any mediastinal lymph nodes removed at the time of operation.

The purposes of hilar and mediastinal LND are accurate staging and the improvement of survival through better local control. The accurate staging is very important because several large-scale randomized trials have shown that postoperative adjuvant chemotherapy can improve the survival after surgery for NSCLC.[5,6] There is no doubt that complete LND is the most accurate way to stage a patient's disease and to determine which patients might benefit from adjuvant therapy. However, the extent of lymph node removal required and the impact of mediastinal lymph node removal on survival are still controversial.

In this article, the impact of LND for NSCLC on the postoperative course, namely, morbidity and survival, is reviewed and discussed.

DEFINITIONS

Although nodal staging of NSCLC should be as accurate as possible, the surgical technique for lymph node assessment varies among countries and centers. It should also be noted that different terms are used to describe these surgical techniques. The definitions for various types of lymph node assessment were recently proposed by the council of the European Society for Thoracic Surgeons.[7]

Lymph Node Biopsy

Only 1 or multiple suspicious lymph nodes are biopsied to prove N1 or N2 disease. No systematic nodal dissection or biopsies are performed. The procedure is performed only to document lymph node metastasis when resection is not justified (**Fig. 1**A).

The author has nothing to disclose.
Department of Thoracic Surgery, Kyoto University Graduate School of Medicine, 54 Shogoin-Kawahara-cho, Sakyo-ku, Kyoto 606-8507, Japan
E-mail address: hdate@kuhp.kyoto-u.ac.jp

Thorac Surg Clin 22 (2012) 239–242
doi:10.1016/j.thorsurg.2011.11.003

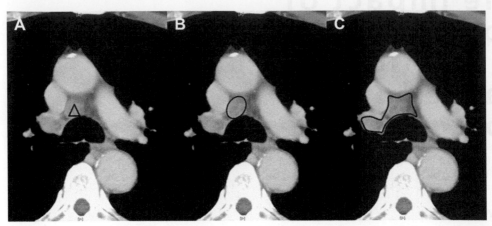

Fig. 1. Differences in the surgical technique for lymph node assessment. (*A*) Lymph node biopsy, (*B*) lymph node sampling, and (*C*) lymph node dissection.

Lymph Node Sampling

One or more lymph nodes are removed without any surrounding tissue, guided by preoperative or intraoperative findings that are thought to be representative (see **Fig. 1**B). Systematic lymph node sampling (LNS) means that a predetermined sampling of the lymph node stations is performed.

Lymph Node Dissection

The mediastinal tissue containing lymph nodes is dissected and removed systematically within anatomic landmarks (see **Fig. 1**C). In other words, all the lymph nodes in the targeted compartment must be completely removed, as a block, together with surrounding adipose tissue.[8] In general, following lobe-specific LND should be performed:

> Right upper and middle lobe: 2R, 4R, and 7
> Right lower lobe: 4R, 7, 8, and 9
> Left upper lobe: 5, 6, and 7
> Left lower lobe: 7, 8, and 9.

COMPARISON BETWEEN LNS AND LND
Mortality and Morbidity

Some surgeons believe that pulmonary resection with LNS is preferable for patients with NSCLC because LND can be associated with significantly increased morbidity, and most recurrences are distant rather than local. In contrast, the standard approach for NSCLC in Japan has been pulmonary resection with systematic LND believing it can achieve better local control with negligible LND related morbidity.

Reasons not to perform LND include prolonging the operation and causing more operative complications such as recurrent nerve injury, chylothorax, bronchial devascularization, increased

lymphatic drainage, and bleeding. Izbicki and colleagues[9] reported that LND did not increase the postoperative mortality or rethoracotomy rate in their prospective randomized trial, but the mean duration of operation increased by 20 minutes. Allen and colleagues[10] reported 30-day operative data from 1,111 patients in a randomized trial comparing LNS and LND. Operative mortality was 2.0% for LNS and 0.8% for LND. Complications occurred in 38% of patients in each group. The investigators also found an increase in operative time by 15 minutes. These studies suggested that LND adds little morbidity to a pulmonary resection for NSCLC, although it requires additional operative time by 15 to 20 minutes.

Survival

So-called stage migration phenomenon between LNS and LND is an important factor that produces bias in retrospective studies. The best evidence is based on prospective randomized trials. Four prospective randomized trials to compare LNS and LND have been performed in Germany,[9,11] Japan,[12] China,[13] and the United States.[10,14,15] Inclusion criteria and methodologies are quite diverse among these studies; therefore, interpretation of each study has to be made carefully.

GERMAN STUDY

> Inclusion criteria: resectable NSCLC based on computed tomography
> Number of patients: LNS (N = 93), LND (N = 76)
> Median follow-up: 47.5 months
> Survival: no difference.

This study is the first prospective randomized trial comparing LNS and LND. A total of 201 patients were recruited for the study, but 32 patients were excluded from analysis because of various reasons.[9,11] Somewhat the LNS group included 17 patients more than the LND group. About 60% of patients were node negative pathologically in each group. There was no difference in survival between LNS and LND ($P = .256$). However, the investigators found a borderline effect on survival ($P = .058$) in patients with pN1 or single-level pN2. They concluded that LND does not influence survival for patients without overt lymph node involvement but might provide benefit for patients with limited lymph node metastases.

JAPANESE STUDY

Inclusion criteria: peripheral NSCLC less than 2 cm, cN0 based on computed tomography

Number of patients: LNS (N = 56), LND (N = 59)

Median follow-up: 65 months

Survival: 5-year survival, LNS (84%) ≒ LND (81%).

This is a small but well-designed study comparing LNS and LND for patients with clinical N0, small (less than 2 cm) NSCLC.[12] Pathologic N2 was found in 14% and 12% of the LNS and LND group, respectively. Survival was similar, and no significant differences in the recurrence rate or survival were observed between the 2 groups. The investigators concluded that clinically evaluated peripheral NSCLCs smaller than 2 cm do not require LND.

CHINESE STUDY

Inclusion criteria: resectable stage I-IIIA based on computed tomography

Number of patients: LNS (N = 264), LND (N = 268)

Median follow-up: more than 5 years

Survival: median survival LND (59 months) >LNS (34 months).

This is a larger trial of 532 patients with clinical stage I-IIIA NSCLC. As compared with the previous study, only about 30% of enrolled patients had stage I disease and 70% of them had nodal involvement.[13] Survival was significantly better in the LND group than in the LNS group. When the 2 groups were compared in subgroups according to pathologic stage, the LND group provided significantly better survival than the LNS group in stages I and IIIA. This study has

been the only randomized trial suggesting the survival benefit of LND.

AMERICAN STUDY

Inclusion criteria[10,14,15]: N0 or nonhilar N1, T1, or T2; all negative lymph nodes after systematic LNS

Number of patients: LNS (N = 498), LND (N = 525)

Median follow-up: 6.5 years

Survival: median survival LNS (8.5 years) ≒ LND (8.1 years).

The American College of Surgeons Oncology Group (ACOSOG) has performed a randomized multi-institutional prospective trial designed to determine whether long-term survival is affected by LND versus LNS at the time of pulmonary resection for NSCLC (ACOSOG Z0030 trial). Of note, this study was not a simple comparison of LNS and LND but designed to assess the efficacy of additional LND when systematic LNS was negative. Systematic LNS was performed at 2R, 4R, 7, and 10R for right-sided tumors and 5, 6, 7, and 10L for left-sided tumors. Occult N2 disease was found in 4% by the additional LND. Survival was similar between LNS and LND groups. There was no difference in local, regional, or distant recurrence between the 2 groups. The investigators concluded that if systematic LNS is negative, LND does not improve survival in patients with early-stage NSCLC.

Although these 4 studies were all prospective, the Chinese study was the only one that showed survival benefit from performing LND, whereas the other 3 studies showed no significant benefit. This difference may be derived from the different inclusion criteria used in each study. One can assume that LND may provide better local control and better survival than LNS only when there is positive lymph node dissected. In other words, when there is no positive lymph node dissected, LND would never be beneficial theoretically. Therefore, how many of the patients enrolled had positive lymph node would affect the outcome of these randomized trials comparing LNS and LND. The ratio of stage I (no lymph node involved) was about 60% in the German study, 30% in the Chinese study, and 80% in the Japanese and American studies. The Japanese and American studies (stage I, 80%) showed no survival benefit of LND, the German study (stage I, 60%) showed borderline effect of LND on survival in patients with pN1 or single-level pN2 disease, and the Chinese study (stage I, 30%) showed significant benefit of LND. In a nonrandomized trial, Keller and colleagues[16] reported the comparison of survival among patients with stage II-IIIA NSCLC who underwent either LNS or LND in the Eastern Cooperative Oncology Group 3590 study. Median survival was 57.5 months for the LND group and 29.2% for the LNS group ($P = .004$).

The ACOSOG Z0030 trial was the largest prospective randomized trial comparing LNS and LND, and it cannot be underestimated. Only 4% of additional patients were found to have positive lymph nodes at LND that were missed at LNS. This study clearly showed that LND does not improve long-term survival in patients with early-stage (T1 or T2, N0, or nonhilar N1) NSCLC who have pathologically negative lymph nodes after rigorous systematic LNS. However, interpretation of this study has to be made carefully because the rigorous systematic LNS performed in this study would not be realistic in a clinical practice in most of the centers and countries. Despite the similar survival between the LNS and LND groups, the investigators of this study still recommended that all patients with resectable NSCLC should undergo LND because the procedure provides the patients with the most accurate staging and the opportunity for effective adjuvant therapy without increasing mortality or morbidity.

REFERENCES

1. Mountain CF. Revisions in the International System for Staging Lung Cancer. Chest 1997;111:1710–7.
2. Naruke T, Suemasu K, Ishikawa S. Lymph node mapping and curability at various levels of metastasis in resected lung cancer. J Thorac Cardiovasc Surg 1978;76:832–9.
3. Martini N, Flehinger BJ, Zaman MB, et al. Prospective study of 445 lung carcinomas with mediastinal lymph node metastases. J Thorac Cardiovasc Surg 1980;80:390–9.
4. Little AG, Rusch VW, Bonner JA, et al. Patterns of surgical care of lung cancer patients. Ann Thorac Surg 2005;80:2051–6.
5. Kato H, Ichinose Y, Ohata M, et al. A randomized trial of adjuvant chemotherapy with uracil-tegafur for adenocarcinoma of the lung. N Engl J Med 2004;350:1713–21.
6. Winton T, Livingston R, Johnson D, et al. Vinorelbine plus cisplatin vs observation in resected non-small-cell lung cancer. N Engl J Med 2005;352:2589–97.
7. Lardinois D, Leyn PD, Schil PV, et al. ESTS guidelines for intraoperative lymph node staging in non-small cell lung cancer. Eur J Cardiothorac Surg 2006;30:787–92.
8. Asamura H. Lymph node dissection for lung cancer. In: Shields TW, Locicero III J, Reed CE, et al, editors. General thoracic surgery. Philadelphia: Lippincott Williams & Wilkins; 2009. p. 1427–33.
9. Izbicki JR, Thetter O, Habekost M, et al. Radical systematic mediastinal lymphadenectomy in non-small cell lung cancer: a randomized controlled trial. Br J Surg 1994;81:229–35.
10. Allen M, Darling GE, Pechet TT, et al. Morbidity and mortality of major pulmonary resections in patients with early-stage lung cancer: initial results of the randomized, prospective ACOSOG Z0030 trial. Ann Thorac Surg 2006;81:1013–20.
11. Izbicki JR, Passlick B, Pantel K, et al. Effectiveness of radical systematic mediastinal lymphadenectomy in patients with resectable non-small cell lung cancer. Ann Surg 1998;227:138–44.
12. Sugi K, Nawata K, Fujita N, et al. Systematic lymph node dissection for clinically diagnosed peripheral non-small-cell lung cancer less than 2 cm in diameter. World J Surg 1998;22:290–5.
13. Wu Y, Huang Z, Wang S, et al. A randomized trial systematic nodal dissection in resectable non-small cell lung cancer. Lung Cancer 2002;36:1–6.
14. Darling GE, Allen MS, Decker PA, et al. Number of lymph nodes harvested from a mediastinal lymphadenectomy: results of the randomized, prospective American College of Surgeons Oncology Group Z0030 trial. Chest 2011;139:1124–9.
15. Darling GE, Allen MS, Decker PA, et al. Randomized trial of mediastinal lymph node sampling versus complete lymphadenectomy during pulmonary resection in the patient with N0 or N1 (less than hilar) non-small cell carcinoma: results of the American College of Surgery Oncology Group Z0030 trial. J Thorac Cardiovasc Surg 2011;141:662–70.
16. Keller SM, Adak S, Wagner H, et al. Mediastinal lymph node dissection improves survival in patients with stage II and IIIa non-small cell lung cancer. Ann Thorac Surg 2000;70:358–66.

The Impact of Chemotherapy on the Lymphatic System in Thoracic Oncology

Antonio Passaro, MD[1],*, Patrizia Trenta, MD[1],
Davide Conte, MD, Giuseppe Campennì, MD,
Angelina De Benedetto, MD, Enrico Cortesi, MD

KEYWORDS

- Non–small cell lung cancer • Adjuvant chemotherapy
- Neoadjuvant chemotherapy • Lymph node

Lung cancer is the leading cause of cancer-related mortality in the United States and Europe. The median 5-year survival rate for patients with non–small cell lung cancer (NSCLC) is about 15%. Relative survival for lung tumors is strongly dependent from stage at diagnosis: 5-years survival is 49%, 16%, and 2% for patients with early, locally advanced, and metastatic disease, respectively.[1,2]

The natural history of lung cancers is influenced by the acquired ability of cancer cells to invade lymphatic and vascular vessels resulting in nodal and distant metastases. In particular, lymphatic spreading generally follows the pulmonary artery branching system: lower lobe lymphatics generally drain to the posterior mediastinum and to the subcarinal nodes; right upper lobe drains to the superior mediastinum; and left upper lobe drains to the anterior and superior mediastinum.

The determination of stage at diagnosis is fundamental in terms of prognostic and therapeutic implications. To plan the best therapeutic strategy, the most important clinical features are the detection of distant metastases and, in nonmetastatic disease, the identification and localization of pathologic thoracic lymph nodes by station. Histologic type, tumor size and location, involvement of pleura, tumor grade, performance status, and biological features are the other cornerstones of prognosis for NSCLC.

Surgery, chemotherapy, target agents, and radiotherapy are the therapeutic options available to treat NSCLC. Surgery is the only really curative treatment choice, but its outcome is still poor, in particular for patients with mediastinal lymph node involvement. Good long-term survival is obtained in stages I and II after pulmonary resection, whereas patient survival after surgery in stage IIIA-N2 is still disappointing. Data from several clinical trials show that in completely resected early stages, the 5-year recurrence rates for patients in stage I, stage II-N0, and stage II-N1 were 16%, 39%, and 46%, respectively.[3,4] On the other side, patients with surgically treated stage IIIA-N2 NSCLC have a 5-year recurrence rate and a 5-year overall survival (OS) rate of 10% to 15%. In particular, patients with bulky mediastinal involvement have a 5-year survival rate of 2% to 5%.[4]

High frequency of distant failure after surgical resection of NSCLC with nodal metastasis suggests that nodal invasion could be considered an indicator of systemic metastasis. Multimodal treatments have been investigated to maximize the gain in survival for patients with metastasis in regional lymph nodes or locally advanced disease.

The authors have no conflict of interest.
Division of Medical Oncology, Sapienza–University of Rome, Viale Regina Elena, 324/00161–Rome, Italy
[1] Both authors contributed equally to this work.
* Corresponding author.
E-mail address: a-passaro@hotmail.it

Thorac Surg Clin 22 (2012) 243–249
doi:10.1016/j.thorsurg.2011.11.002
1547-4127/12/$ – see front matter © 2012 Elsevier Inc. All rights reserved.

Presurgical staging is extremely important to select the correct therapeutic strategy in a patient with newly diagnosed NSCLC, but no single examination is sufficient alone to determine both lymph nodal status and the presence of distant metastases at the moment.

Several radiologic investigations such as computed tomography (CT), bone scan, positron emission tomography (PET) or magnetic resonance imaging of the brain are performed for initial assessment. However, these noninvasive techniques, performed for preoperative staging, seem to be still imperfect for the correct evaluation of thoracic nodal involvement. Invasive surgical procedures, such as mediastinoscopy, are the gold standard for the correct evaluation of lymph nodal status. Mediastinoscopy can help clinicians to select patients eligible for surgery from those who will receive only a palliative treatment; above all, it should be mandatory to select patients with a locally advanced disease who could benefit from a preoperative downstaging induction treatment.[5,6]

After surgery, most patients develop regional or distant metastases, in particular those with pathologic nodal involvement. Several randomized adjuvant/neoadjuvant trials, using chemotherapy and/or radiotherapy investigated the possibility to improve the outcome of patients with lung cancer by increasing their OS. Use of postoperative chemotherapy in patients with resected NSCLC has been evaluated in several randomized controlled trials and meta-analyses, and a 5-year absolute benefit of about 5% was obtained with cisplatin-based doublet regimens.[7] On the other side, postoperative radiotherapy (PORT) showed detrimental effects in patients with pathologic stage I/II and N0-N1 disease, with an 18% relative increase of the death risk for patients who received PORT compared with those who underwent surgery alone (hazard ratio [HR], 1.18, $P = .002$). In resected stage IIIA-N2 disease, this adverse effect is controversial. Although some studies suggest that PORT can improve local control for patients with node-positive lung cancer who have undergone surgical resection, it remains unclear whether PORT can really improve survival. Postoperative chemoradiotherapy for stage IIIA-N2 NSCLC has been evaluated in 5 randomized trials versus radiation following surgical resection; only 1 trial reported a disease-free survival gain by adding chemotherapy to radiotherapy, but no trial reported improvement in OS. No difference in local control or survival was observed in 3 trials evaluating platinum-based chemotherapy followed by surgery versus combined platinum-based chemoradiotherapy alone in IIIA-N2 diseases, but those studies were small and with a limited enrollment.[8]

Radiation and chemoradiotherapy have also been investigated as exclusive treatments for unresectable stage IIIA-N2 NSCLC; both treatments are not curative, and they are performed for a long-term survival benefit and palliation of symptoms.

Neoadjuvant chemotherapy in resectable node-negative and node-positive lung cancers has also been investigated, with controversial results. This therapy aims to reduce tumor size, facilitate surgical resection, eradicate micrometastases, and improve tolerability. Of particular interest is the possible role that preoperative chemotherapy could play in a particularly heterogeneous group of patients, those with stage IIIA with resectable or potentially resectable N2 tumor.

It is clear that nodal thoracic involvement is the principal clinical feature that influences the prognosis of patients with nonmetastatic NSCLC. The aim of the present analysis is to evaluate if and how a medical treatment such as chemotherapy, given before or after surgery, can improve the outcome and reduce cancer-related mortality of both patients with node-negative and node-positive NSCLC.

IMPACT OF ADJUVANT TREATMENT ON THORACIC LYMPH NODE INVOLVEMENT

Adjuvant chemotherapy has been explored with the goal of eliminating occult metastases and reducing the risk of recurrence. Adjuvant trials (the first- and second-generation ones) have sometimes shown controversial results, but, in 2008, the Lung Adjuvant Cisplatin Evaluation (LACE) collaborative group published a meta-analysis based on data from the 5 largest trials of cisplatin-based adjuvant chemotherapy (Adjuvant Lung Cancer Project Italy [ALPI], Adjuvant Navelbine International Trialist Association [ANITA], International Adjuvant Lung Cancer Trial [IALT], Big Lung Trial [BLT], and JBR.10) that confirmed a 5-year absolute survival benefit of about 5.4% for postoperative chemotherapy for stage II and III disease[7] that was sufficient to recommend adjuvant cisplatin-based treatment as part of clinical routine practice.[9]

When radical surgery is performed (lobectomy or pneumonectomy and lymphadenectomy), the nodal pathologic status is of great importance to determine if patients will benefit or not from an adjuvant treatment and how much relevant is this benefit, as can be deduced from the subgroup analysis of principal adjuvant studies. Some differences can be found if the results of the principal trials are analyzed stage by stage (I, II, and IIIA) and, in particular, according to nodal pathologic status (pN0 vs pN1-2 disease).

The only 2 adjuvant cisplatin-based trials (ALPI and IALT) including stage IA NSCLC agree about the detrimental effect that chemotherapy has for these patients,[10,11] with an overall HR for OS of 1.4 (95% confidence interval [CI], 0.95–2.06).[7]

If chemotherapy should have a role in adjuvant treatment of stage IB cancer (referring to the 6th edition of TNM) is still an open question because of the controversial data derived from clinical trials. After a follow-up of 76 months, ANITA trial established lack of survival advantage from adjuvant chemotherapy for all patients with pN0 stage I disease with an HR of 1.14 (95% CI, 0.83–1.57).[12] Similar data come from long-term follow-up of JBR.10 study,[13] IALT trial,[5] and LACE meta-analyses.[7] However, CALGB [Cancer and Leukemia Group B] 9633 study expressly created to test adjuvant treatment with carboplatin and paclitaxel in high-risk node-negative disease (stage IB) gives some points of reflection. Although preliminarily finding of the study encouraged chemotherapy use, with a surprising HR for OS of 0.62 (90% CI, 0.44–0.89, P = .14), mature data after a longer follow-up (74 months) showed a 17% reduction of the risk of death for the chemotherapy group but without statistical significance (HR, 0.83; 90% CI, 0.64 to 1.08; P = .125). The small number of enrolled patients probably let the study to be underpowered to detect survival differences between the 2 arms. Despite this, an unplanned subgroup analysis of the same trial showed a 31% reduction of the risk of death for patients treated with chemotherapy whose tumors were 4 cm and larger (HR, 0.69; 90% CI, 0.48–0.99; P = .043), with a similar advantage for disease-free survival also. A trend toward inferior OS and disease-free survival for the chemotherapy group was observed for those patients with pT of 4 cm or less, pN0.[14] This could mean that only smaller pN0 NSCLCs do not benefit of adjuvant treatment.

Anyway, whether patients with stage IB tumors should be treated with systemic adjuvant chemotherapy is still an open question. The Union for International Cancer Control seventh TNM classification reclassifies pT2 pN0 tumors larger than 5 cm in diameter as stage IIA instead of IB; this could partially solve this controversy.

On the other side, the positive role of adjuvant chemotherapy for node-positive disease seems to be well established, but some differences between pN1 and pN2 NSCLCs can be found in terms of magnitude of the absolute benefit if clinical trial results are deeply analyzed. For example, according to the ANITA trial, patients with a greater node involvement would benefit more from chemotherapy; HR for OS for pN1 disease is 0.67 (0.47–0.94), whereas it is 0.60 (0.44–0.82) for patients with pN2 NSCLC. In particular, in patients with pathologic stage IIIA, the study showed an improvement in survival of 16%.[12]

IALT subgroup analyses show a real survival advantage only for pN2 disease,[5] whereas the principal meta-analyses of second-generation cisplatin-based adjuvant trials (LACE) did not find any difference in survival advantage between stage II and III NSCLC (both HR, 0.83 [0.73–0.95] P = .04).[7]

It seems clear that the impact of adjuvant treatment is strictly influenced by nodal status; for pN0 little tumors chemotherapy should be detrimental, whereas available data seem to suggest that benefit maximizes when there is a greater nodal involvement. Adjuvant radiotherapy, allowed in some of those trials, could have played an important role in influencing this survival advantage, most of all for pN2 disease.

IMPACT OF NEOADJUVANT TREATMENT ON THORACIC LYMPH NODE INVOLVEMENT

Neoadjuvant chemotherapy generally gives some important advantages in the management of non-metastatic tumors because it allows an early control on systemic micrometastasis, giving the possibility to reduce tumor volume, facilitating surgical approach, and granting a better compliance to chemotherapy, with a generally higher dose intensity. Moreover, it is a way to test chemotherapy efficacy in vivo. On the other hand, possible toxicities and consequent delaying of surgery should sometimes be detrimental. Despite this theoretical rationale, the efficacy of neoadjuvant treatment of early-stage disease is still not so clear; the greatest part of individual trials found a trend over a survival benefit for neoadjuvant therapy that did not reach the statistical significance, probably because of the underpowering of the individual studies or the contamination of the outcome by the use of adjuvant therapy in some of them. For that reason, neoadjuvant medical treatment is still considered an experimental approach for early-stage disease.[15]

Available data demonstrate some differences in the impact of neoadjuvant chemotherapy according to nodal clinical involvement. In 2002, Depierre and colleagues[16] published a phase III clinical trial in which 355 patients with resectable (IB-IIIA) NSCLC were randomized to 2 cycles of induction chemotherapy (and 2 more cycles after surgery) or surgery alone. Despite the impressive differences in 3- and 4-year survivals observed in favor of preoperative approach, survival advantage was significant only for cN0 (not T1) to cN1 disease (HR, 0.68; 95% CI, 0.49–0.96) and not for patients with cN2 disease (HR, 1.04; 95% CI, 0.68–1.60). Despite these impressive results, larger trials did not confirm the benefit of neoadjuvant chemotherapy for patients with cN2 disease. In the investigators' trial, there was no statistically significant gain in survival for patients affected by NSCLC stage IIIA-N2 (HR, 1.04) receiving preoperative treatment.

The SWOG (Southwest Oncology Group) 9900 trial of neoadjuvant chemotherapy excluded clinical N2 disease. The advantage in OS and progression-free survival of administering treatment based on carboplatin/paclitaxel before surgery did not join the statistical significance (probably because of the lower than expected accrual), but cN0 disease seems to benefit more from preoperative treatment with an HR of 1.43 (95% CI, 1.05–1.96; $P = .025$) in favor of lower stages.[17]

Of particular interest are the role and effective benefit of neoadjuvant chemotherapy in potentially resectable stage IIIA-N2 NSCLC.

In 1994, Rosell and colleagues[18] published the results of a phase III randomized trial examining the possible benefit of preoperative chemotherapy for 60 patients diagnosed with stage IIIA NSCLC. Patients were randomly assigned to receive either surgery alone or 3 courses of neoadjuvant chemotherapy, given intravenously at 3-week intervals, followed by surgery. All patients received mediastinal radiation after surgical resection. Median survival in the group receiving induction chemotherapy was 26 months compared with 8 months in those treated with surgery alone ($P<.001$); 5-years survival was 17% for patients treated with neoadjuvant chemotherapy versus 0% for those treated with surgical resection only.[18]

In the same year, the results of another randomized phase III trial of preoperative chemotherapy was published by Roth and colleagues[19] from MD Anderson Cancer Center. In this trial, 60 patients with potentially resectable clinical stage IIIA NSCLC were randomized to receive preoperative chemotherapy and then surgery or surgery alone. Median survival time was 21 months in patients treated with neoadjuvant chemotherapy and 14 months for other patients not receiving medical treatment ($P = .056$). The 5-year survivals for the perioperative chemotherapy group and the surgery-alone group were 36% and 15%, respectively.

Despite these impressive results, larger trials did not confirm the benefit of neoadjuvant chemotherapy for patients with cN2 disease.

In addition to these studies, 2 meta-analyses explored the role of induction chemotherapy in patients with NSCLC with or without lymph node involvements showing a better effect of treatment of more advanced stages. In the first study,

Berghmans and colleagues[20] analyzed data from 6 randomized trials, published between 1990 and 2003, based on a comparison of induction chemotherapy followed by surgery versus surgery alone for a total of 590 patients. Only in 4 of these trials, patients with stage III NSCLC only were included. The results of this meta-analysis showed the greatest efficacy of induction chemotherapy in the subgroup of patients with clinical resectable stage IIIA-N2 NSCLC at initial workup with an HR of 0.65 (95% CI, 0.41–1.04; $P = .02$) for survival. The second meta-analysis published in 2006 by Burdett and colleagues,[21] based on 12 trials, including 988 patients, showed improved survival for patients treated with preoperative chemotherapy with an HR of 0.82 (95% CI, 0.69–0.97), a 5-years absolute benefit of 6% (similar to adjuvant therapy), and increasing OS across all stages of disease from 14% to 20% at 5 years. This benefit seems to increase for higher stages (and consequently for higher nodal involvement): stage IA, +4%; stage IB, +6%; and stage II-III, +7%.

Furthermore, the rate of nodal response to induction chemotherapy and the clearance of mediastinal lymph nodes in cN2 operable tumors, in particular, have been hypothesized to be also a prognostic factor. Although many studies evaluate the effect in survival of adjuvant and/or neoadjuvant chemotherapy, there are only a few trials that assessed the impact of chemotherapy on lymph node downstaging before surgery.

In 2000, Bueno and colleagues[22] published the results of their study that determined the predictive value of nodal status at resection in regard to long-term outcome of patients undergoing neoadjuvant therapy and resection for stage IIIA-N2–positive NSCLC. In this study, 103 patients were enrolled (44 woman and 59 men); of these, 55 patients had adenocarcinoma, 33 had squamous cell carcinoma, 9 had undifferentiated NSCLC, 5 had large cell cancer, and 1 patient had adenosquamous carcinoma. All the patients enrolled in this study had an involvement of lymphatic system; 57 patients had paratracheal lymph node involvement, 30 had subcarinal lymph node involvement, 29 had aortopulmonary window or subaortic lymph node involvement, and 2 had pulmonary ligament lymph node involvement. After induction chemotherapy, 2 patients showed a complete pathologic response with downstaging to T0N0. In 18 patients the disease downstaged to stage N0 and in 21 to N1, whereas 37 patients remained N2 positive at resection. Before surgery, 74 patients received an additional treatment; 58 patients received radiotherapy, 14 concomitant chemotherapy and radiation therapy, and 2 chemotherapy alone. The results showed a 5-year survival of 17.5%, with a median survival of 17.8 months. In a subgroup of 29 patients in whom the disease downstaged to N0, the 5-year survival was 35.8%, with a median survival of 21.3 months. The freedoms from recurrence at 12 and 24 months were 71% (CI, 51%–85%) and 43% (CI, 25%–60%), respectively, for patients who were node negative at the time of resection. The freedom from recurrence at the same time intervals for patients who were node positive at the time of resection was significantly lower (43% [CI, 31%–55%] and 22% [CI 12%–33%]). The results of this interesting trial revealed that there were 2 significant and independent factors associated with improved cancer-free survival in these patients: freedom from nodal disease at resection and histology other than adenocarcinoma.[22]

A Belgian experience including 92 patients with pathology-confirmed operable cN2 NSCLC showed a downstaging (ypN0-1) of mediastinal lymph nodes in 43% of the sample treated with induction chemotherapy. A trend for better survival in those patients was observed, with a 5-years survival of 49% versus 27% in patients with persistent N2 disease ($P = .095$). Maybe, this was not significant because patients with persistent N2 disease underwent radiotherapy. Moreover, in patients with pN2 disease, a significant difference in 5-years survival was found between those with single-level versus multilevel nodal involvement (37% vs 7.1%; $P<.005$).[23] Multilevel ypN2 and ypN3 had been identified as negative prognostic factors in previous reporting,[24,25] and recent series confirm a significant difference in survival between patients with and without downstaged mediastinal lymph nodes after induction chemotherapy as if the sterilization of the mediastinum could be an important predictor of good outcome.[26]

COMMENT

The therapeutic strategy of NSCLC has undergone deep changes over the past year with the introduction of new chemotherapeutic and target agents in clinical practice. Despite considerable progress over the last decade, the prognosis of this disease remains severe with a 5-year survival rate of 16% to 49% for radically resected cases and about 2% for inoperable cases.[1]

Approximately 26% to 44% of patients with NSCLC present mediastinal lymph node involvement at diagnosis, which is the most important prognostic factor in early-stage NSCLC, and multimodal treatments show a better influence on survival than surgery alone in patients with lymph node metastatic disease. Based on currently available data, adjuvant chemotherapy is considered a standard treatment in patients with stage II-IIIA tumor radically operated who recovered after surgery in good general condition and do not have contraindications to the use of platinum with approximately a 5-years survival of 5%.[11] At present, platinum-based doublet as adjuvant chemotherapy is recommended for patients with completely resected stage II and IIIA, for no more than 4 cycles and should be initiated no later than 2 months by surgery,[27] for the high recurrence of metastatic disease (about 60%–70%).[28,29] The poor survival rates after surgery alone in cN2 disease has led to designing protocols with neoadjuvant therapy before nonsurgical treatment (radiotherapy and/or chemotherapy), especially to convert to surgery "unresectable" tumor, eradicate any micrometastases, and improve long-term survival of resectable cN2 NSCLC. Andre and colleagues[28] investigated the heterogeneity of mediastinal lymph node involvement in 702 patients treated with surgical resection of N2 NSCLC. In these patients, the 5-year survivals rate varied according to N2 characteristics: one level involvement with microscopic disease (34%), multiple level lymph nodes with microscopic disease (11%), single-level clinically apparent disease (8%), and multilevel clinically apparent disease (3%). Neoadjuvant or induction chemotherapy offers different potential advantages compared with adjuvant chemotherapy, such as improved compliance, drug delivery, early control of micrometastases, and shrink tumor volume before surgery, thus allowing for more conservative and possibly complete cancer resection.[29] At present, the role of induction chemotherapy remains ill defined, but it is emerging in technically resectable stage IIIA-N2 disease.[20,21] Patients with cN3 disease are not thought to be candidates for surgery and they are treated with concurrent chemotherapy/radiation therapy. In patients with stage IIIA - N2 NSCLC the 5-years survival is from 20% to 30% compared with 5% to 10% for surgery alone.[16] The disease in patients with documented pathologic mediastinal lymph node disease will be found at surgery to be downstaged after multimodality therapy in approximately 45% to 65% of the cases.[22,30,31] Mediastinal clearance and complete resection of tumor in these patients has been associated with a 3-year survival of 53% to 61%, compared with 11% to 18% for those without mediastinal clearance. These evidences suggest that mediastinal nodal sterilization is the strongest predictor of long-term survival, and it could be a surrogate marker for eradication of distant chemotherapy-sensitive micrometastases.[32,33] Surgical resection should be avoided in patients after induction therapy who have definite biopsy-proven residual tumor in the mediastinal nodes, and definitive chemotherapy/radiotherapy treatment should be preferred.

Based on the contradictory results and limitations of phase 2 and 3 clinical trials, the benefit of induction chemotherapy in patients with resectable stage IB-II-IIIA selected disease remains uncertain, and additional studies are warranted to further address this issue.

SUMMARY

Pathologic lymph node involvement is an important prognostic factor for patients with NSCLC. Several trials showed that lung cancer resection combined with complete lymph node dissection is associated with a modest improvement in survival. In these cases, chemotherapy in adjuvant or neoadjuvant settings can improve the survival rate. The role of chemotherapy in patients with lymph node involvement depends from stage at diagnosis. In stage II and IIIA, different studies indicate that cisplatin-based adjuvant chemotherapy improves 5-year survival, whereas the use of adjuvant chemotherapy in stage I remains controversial. Induction chemotherapy presents different benefits over adjuvant chemotherapy, particularly for stage IIIA-N2 disease. In these patients, neoadjuvant chemotherapy should be considered the standard of care, to shrink tumor size and eradicate micrometastases, with a better tolerability than adjuvant treatment. Despite these encouraging results, further studies are needed to define the role of preoperative and postoperative chemotherapy in NSCLC early stage with lymph node involvement. Although clinical and pathologic prognostic factors drive the selection of the best treatment, in patients with lymph node involvements, a multimodal approach between surgery, chemotherapy, and radiotherapy is needed not only to improve survival but also to keep a good quality of life.

REFERENCES

1. Jemal A, Siegel R, Ward E, et al. Cancer statistics, 2010. CA Cancer J Clin 2010;60(5):277–300.
2. Ries L, Eisner M, Kosary C, et al. Cancer statistics review, 1975-2002. Bethesda (MD): National Cancer Institute; 2005. Available at: http://seer.cancer.gov/. Accessed August 13, 2010.
3. Martini N, Bains MS, Burt ME, et al. Incidence of local recurrence and second primary tumors in resected stage I lung cancer. J Thorac Cardiovasc Surg 1995;109(1):120–9.
4. Maeda R, Yoshida J, Ishii G, et al. Poor prognostic factors in patients with stage IB non small cell lung cancer according to the seventh edition TNM classification. Chest 2011;139(4):855–61.
5. Webb WR, Gatsonis C, Zerhouni EA, et al. CT and MR imaging in staging non-small cell bronchogenic carcinoma: report of the Radiologic Diagnostic Oncology Group. Radiology 1991;178(3):705–13.
6. Toloza EM, Harpole L, McCrory DC. Noninvasive staging of non-small cell lung cancer: a review of the current evidence. Chest 2003;123(Suppl 1): 137S–46S.
7. Pignon JP, Tribodet H, Scagliotti GV, et al. Lung adjuvant cisplatin evaluation: a pooled analysis by the LACE Collaborative Group. J Clin Oncol 2008; 26(21):3552–9.
8. PORT Meta-analysis Trialists Group. Postoperative radiotherapy for non-small cell lung cancer. Cochrane Database Syst Rev 2005;2:CD002142.
9. Crino' L, Weder W, Van Meerbeeck J, et al. Early stage and locally advanced (non-metastatic) non-small-cell lung cancer: ESMO Clinical Practice Guidelines for diagnosis, treatment and follow-up. Ann Oncol 2010;21(Suppl 5):v103–15.
10. Scagliotti GV, Fossati R, Torri V, et al. Randomized study of adjuvant chemotherapy for completely resected stage I, II, or IIIA non–small-cell lung cancer. J Natl Cancer Inst 2003;95(19):1453–61.
11. The International Adjuvant Lung Cancer Trial Collaborative Group. Cisplatin-based adjuvant chemotherapy in patients with completely resected nonsmall cell lung cancer. N Engl J Med 2004;350: 351–60.
12. Douillard JY, Rosell R, De Lena M, et al. Adjuvant vinorelbine plus cisplatin versus observation in patients with completely resected stage IB–IIIA non-small-cell lung cancer (Adjuvant Navelbine International Trialist Association [ANITA]): a randomised controlled trial. Lancet Oncol 2006;7:719–27.
13. Butts CA, Ding K, Seymour L, et al. Randomized phase III trial of vinorelbine plus cisplatin compared with observation in completely resected stage IB and II non–small-cell lung cancer: updated survival analysis of JBR-10. J Clin Oncol 2010;28(1):29–34.
14. Strauss GM, Herndon JE, Maddaus MA, et al. Adjuvant paclitaxel plus carboplatin compared with observation in stage IB non–small-cell lung cancer: CALGB 9633 with the Cancer and Leukemia Group B, Radiation Therapy Oncology Group, and North Central Cancer Treatment Group Study Groups. J Clin Oncol 2008;26(31):5043–51.
15. De Marinis F, Gebbia V, De Petris L. Neoadjuvant chemotherapy for stage IIIA-N2 non-small cell lung cancer. Ann Oncol 2005;16(Suppl 4):iv116–22.
16. Depierre A, Milleron B, Moro-Sibilot D, et al. Preoperative chemotherapy followed by surgery compared with primary surgery in resectable stage I (except T1N0), II, and IIIa non-small-cell lung cancer. J Clin Oncol 2002;20(1):247.

17. Pisters K, Vallie'res E, Crowley J, et al. Surgery with or without preoperative paclitaxel and carboplatin in early-stage non–small-cell lung cancer: Southwest Oncology Group Trial S9900, an intergroup, randomized, phase III trial. J Clin Oncol 2010;28:1843–9.

18. Rosell R, Gómez-Codina J, Camps C, et al. A randomized trial comparing preoperative chemotherapy plus surgery with surgery alone in patients with non-small-cell lung cancer. N Engl J Med 1994;330(3):153–8.

19. Roth JA, Fossella F, Komaki R, et al. A randomized trial comparing perioperative chemotherapy and surgery with surgery alone in resectable stage IIIA non-small-cell lung cancer. J Natl Cancer Inst 1994;86(9):673–80.

20. Berghmans T, Paesmans M, Meert AP, et al. Survival improvement in resectable non-small cell lung cancer with (neo)adjuvant chemotherapy: results of a meta-analysis of the literature. Lung Cancer 2005;49:13–23.

21. Burdett S, Stewart L, Rydzewska L, et al. A systematic review and meta-analysis of the literature: chemotherapy and surgery versus surgery alone in non-small cell lung cancer. J Thorac Oncol 2006;1:611–21.

22. Bueno R, Richards WG, Swanson SJ, et al. Nodal stage after induction therapy for stage IIIA lung cancer determines patient survival. Ann Thorac Surg 2000;70(6):1826–31.

23. Decaluwé H, De Leyn P, Vansteenkiste J, et al. Surgical multimodality treatment for baseline resectable stage IIIA-N2 non-small cell lung cancer. Degree of mediastinal lymph node involvement and impact on survival. Eur J Cardiothorac Surg 2009;36:433–9.

24. Rusch VW, Crowley J, Giroux DJ, et al. The IASLC lung cancer staging project: proposals for the revision of the N descriptors in the forthcoming seventh edition of the TNM classification for lung cancer. J Thorac Oncol 2007;2(7):603–12.

25. Paul S, Mirza F, Port JL, et al. Survival of patients with clinical stage IIIA non–small cell lung cancer after induction therapy: age, mediastinal downstaging, and extent of pulmonary resection as independent predictors. J Thorac Cardiovasc Surg 2011;141(1):48–58.

26. Scagliotti GV, Novello S. Current status of adjuvant chemotherapy in NSCLC. Ann Oncol 2006;17:62–3.

27. Betticher DC, Hsu Schmitz SF, Totsch M, et al. Prognostic factors affecting long-term outcomes in patients with resected stage IIIA pN2 non-small-cell lung cancer: 5-year follow-up of a phase II study. Br J Cancer 2006;94(8):1099.

28. Andre F, Grunenwald D, Pignon JP, et al. Survival of patients with resected N2 non-small-cell lung cancer: evidence for a subclassification and implications. J Clin Oncol 2000;18(16):2981.

29. Albain KS, Rusch VW, Crowley JJ, et al. Concurrent cisplatin/etoposide plus chest radiotherapy followed by surgery for stages IIIA (N2) and IIIB non-small-cell lung cancer: mature results of Southwest Oncology Group phase II study 8805. J Clin Oncol 1995;13:1880–92.

30. Pass HI, Pogrebniak HW, Steinberg SM, et al. Randomized trial of neoadjuvant therapy for lung cancer: interim analysis. Ann Thorac Surg 1992;53:992–8.

31. Betticher DC, Hsu Schmitz SF, Totsch M, et al. Mediastinal lymph node clearance after docetaxel-cisplatin neoadjuvant chemotherapy is prognostic of survival in patients with stage IIIA pN2 non-small-cell lung cancer: a multicenter phase II trial. J Clin Oncol 2003;21:1752–9.

32. De WM, Hendriks J, Lauwers P, et al. Nodal status at repeat mediastinoscopy determines survival in non-small-cell lung cancer with mediastinal nodal involvement, treated by induction therapy. Eur J Cardiothorac Surg 2006;29(2):240.

33. Port JL, Korst RJ, Lee PC, et al. Surgical resection for residual N2 disease after induction chemotherapy. Ann Thorac Surg 2005;79(5):1686.

Index

Note: Page numbers of article titles are in **boldface** type.

Thorac Surg Clin 22 (2012) 251–255
doi:10.1016/S1547-4127(12)00010-2
1547-4127/12/$ – see front matter © 2012 Elsevier Inc. All rights reserved.

thoracic.theclinics.com